MECHANICS AND ENERGETICS OF THE MYOCARDIUM

BASIC SCIENCE FOR THE CARDIOLOGIST

1. B. Swynghedauw (ed.): *Molecular Cardiology for the Cardiologist*. Second Edition. 1998 ISBN: 0-7923-8323-0
2. B. Levy, A. Tedgui (eds.): *Biology of the Arterial Wall*. 1999 ISBN 0-7923-8458-X
3. M.R. Sanders, J.B. Kostis (eds): *Molecular Cardiology in Clinical Practice*. 1999. ISBN 0-7923-8602-7
4. B. Ostadal, F. Kolar (eds.): *Cardiac Ischemia: From Injury to Protection*. 1999 ISBN 0-7923-8642-6
5. H. Schunkert, G.A.J. Riegger (eds.): *Apoptosis in Cardiac Biology*. 1999 ISBN 0-7923-8648-5
6. A. Malliani, (ed.): *Principles of Cardiovascular Neural Regulation in Health and Disease*. 2000 ISBN 0-7923-7775-3
7. P. Benlian : Ge*netics of Dyslipidemia*. 2001 ISBN 0-7923-7362-6
8. D. Young : *Role of Potassium in Preventive Cardiovascular Medicine*. 2001 ISBN 0-7923-7376-6
9. E. Carmeliet, J. Vereecke : *Cardiac Cellular Electrophysiology*. 2002 ISBN 0-7923-7544-0
10. Ch. Holubarsch : Mechanics and Energetics of the Myocardium. 2002 ISBN 0-7923-7570-X

KLUWER ACADEMIC PUBLISHERS - DORDRECHT/BOSTON/LONDON

MECHANICS AND ENERGETICS OF THE MYOCARDIUM

by

Christian J. F. Holubarsch
Department of Cardiology & Angiology
Medizinische Klinik
University of Freiburg
Germany

KLUWER ACADEMIC PUBLISHERS
Boston / Dordrecht / London

Distributors for North, Central and South America:
Kluwer Academic Publishers
101 Philip Drive
Assinippi Park
Norwell, Massachusetts 02061 USA
Telephone (781) 871-6600
Fax (781) 681-9045
E-Mail <kluwer@wkap.com>

Distributors for all other countries:
Kluwer Academic Publishers Group
Distribution Centre
Post Office Box 322
3300 AH Dordrecht, THE NETHERLANDS
Telephone 31 78 6392 392
Fax 31 78 6546 474
E-Mail <services@wkap.nl>

Electronic Services <http://www.wkap.nl>

Library of Congress Cataloging-in-Publication Data

Holubarsch, Ch.
Mechanics and energetics of the myocardium / by Christian Holubarsch.
p. ; cm. – (Basic science for the cardiologist ; 10)
Co-authors: M. Philipp Schröder and Helge Möllmann
Includes bibliographical references and index.
ISBN 0-7923-7570-X (alk. Paper)
1. Myocardium-Physiology. 2.Myocardium-Pathophysiology. 3.Heart-Contraction.
I. Schröder, M. Philipp. II. Möllmann, Helge. III. Title. IV. Series.
[DNLM: 1. Myocardium. 2. Heart—physiology. WG H758m 2002]
QP113.2 .H65 2002
612.1'7– dc21

2001050353

Printed on acid-free paper. Printed in the United States of America

TABLE OF CONTENTS

LIST OF CONTRIBUTORS

Christian J. F. Holubarsch
Department of Cardiology & Angiology
Medizinische Klinik
University of Freiburg
Hugstetter Strasse 55
79106 Freiburg
Germany

Co-authors: M. Philipp Schröder and Helge Möllmann

PREFACE

During several decades of this century, the classical physiological studies on the cardiovascular system have greatly improved our knowledge on the function of this system under normal and pathological conditions. This knowledge was the basis of the breakthrough for diagnostic techniques like the Swan-Ganz catheter, coronary arteriography, left and right heart biopsies, and invasive measurements of contractility as well as therapeutic tools including aortocoronary bypass surgery, percutanous transluminal coronary angioplasty and a broad field of pharmacological interventions for the whole spectrum of cardiovascular diseases, especially chronic heart failure.

It was during the last decade that the scientific world focused much more on the extremely fast evolution of molecular biology of the cardiovascular system so that cardiovascular physiology seemed to become less important. Regarding the myocardium, molecular alterations of important functional proteins (phenotype changes) as well as signal transduction pathways of contractility and cardiac growth have been elucidated. Especially, with the help of transgenic animals, the functional importance of a number of genes has undoubtedly been proven.

In these days, cardiovascular physiology is regaining its importance, because only the synopsis between molecular alterations and mechanics and energetics of the myocardium can help to understand myocardial function of the normal and the diseased heart. Only the relationship between gene expression and its functional consequences regarding mechanics and energetics may help in developing both modern pharmacological compounds and future gene therapy.

It was my goal to provide a review on "Mechanics and Energetics of the Myocardium", especially for younger researchers that are interested in molecular biology and physiology of the cardiovascular system and need an overview on this broad field with respect to methodological approaches as well as proven facts. Certainly, I am aware of the fact that this review may not cover all physiological and pathophysiological aspects. I will rather concentrate on those subjects with which the authors are most familiar.

I thought it might be useful to include some historical aspects. Therefore, two chapters are antecedent to the manuscript: Chapter I deals with our understanding of the Frank-Starling mechanism, i.e., the length-dependency of contractile force in normal and diseased states. Furthermore, the study of myocardial energetics is fundamentally based on the use of thermopiles in order to measure the heat liberated by a skeletal or cardiac muscle preparation. This latter chapter was chosen, because my own scientific career was profoundly connected with experimental work in this special field which allowed me to meet well-known cardiac and skeletal muscle physiologists from all over the world, personally.

The chapters III to X describe in great detail the various approaches used to investigate mechanics and energetics of the myocardium. Starting with papillary muscle (chapter III) and the myothermal method (chapter IV), we afterwards discuss skinned fiber experiments (chapter V) as well as single cell experiments (chapter VII). Chapter VI handles the frequency response method and chapter VIII the passive elastic properties of cardiac muscle. Finally, chapter IX and X deal with oxygen consumption measurement of whole hearts in vitro and in vivo.

Each chapter is constructed in the following way: An introduction gives some historical aspects and provides some fundamental understanding of the research. It is followed by a method section that critically describes the methodological approaches in great detail as well as difficulties, advantages and disadvantages, and general problems of the specific method. In the results section the most important findings are demonstrated by the use of either original illustrations or schematic drawings or tables differentiating especially between data obtained in animal and human myocardium.

In the future, more molecular biology research will provide a better understanding for the observed mechanic and energetic changes in hypertrophy and failure and will certainly open new therapeutic strategies by developing new pharmacological and genetic tools for the normalization of gene expression.

Acknowledgments:
The help of Mr. Stefan Wollner regarding the composition of chapters and the integration of figures is greatly appreciated.

This book is dedicated to the former Director of the Department of Physiology, University of Tuebingen, Germany, Prof. Dr. Ruthard Jacob, who was my first and most important teacher in Physiology – on occasion of his 75th birthday.

Prof. Dr. Christian J. F. Holubarsch
Freiburg, November 12th, 2000

I. HISTORICAL ASPECTS: THE FRANK-STARLING MECHANISM

To guarantee sufficient blood supply to all organs during a life of a mammalian organism, arterial blood pressure has to be controlled permanently within narrow physiological ranges. This is achieved by several biological systems that regulate peripheral circulation as well as a number of mechanisms influencing the vigor of the heart beat. The following mechanisms influence cardiac contractile performance in concert: (1) The Frank-Starling mechanism [1,2]; (2) the Bowditch-Treppe [3]; (3) the sympathetic and parasympathetic nervous system [4]; and (4) some vasoactive hormones (angiotensins [5,6], endothelin [7,8,9]). The preload or muscle-length dependency of cardiac contractile performance has been called Frank-Starling mechanism (FSM), because the German physiologist Otto Frank was the first who gave a profound description and an exact definition of this fundamental physiological phenomenon already in 1895: "...this finding falls under the above mentioned law established by Fick [10] for skeletal muscle and by me for the heart muscle: The maximal tension of isometric contraction at first increases with augmentation of the initial length (or initial tension [end-diastolic]). It is inherent in the above law that the absolute strength is represented by the maximal tensions of the first part of the isometric family curves" (Figure 1).

During the last 100 years, plenty of evidence has been found that this mechanism is not only present in animal and human myocardium, but plays a fundamental role in the regulation of the heart's pumping function and contributes to maintenance of circulation in vivo during rest and exercise. Interestingly, a mixture of molecular structures or mechanisms has been proposed to be responsible for the law of Frank and Starling.

However, during the past 100 years, the existence or importance of the FSM has been questioned and its physiological role has been discussed controversially, especially in the light of other more potent control mechanisms of myocardial contractile performance. Quite recently and more importantly, an attenuation or even a complete loss of the FSM has been postulated for end-stage failing human myocardium [11,12].

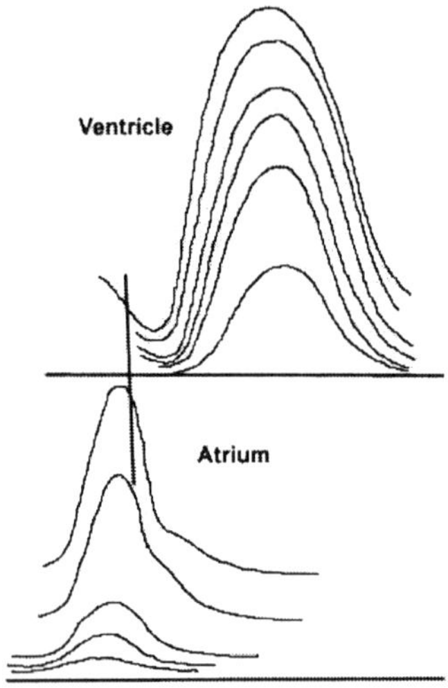

Figure 1: Family of isometric curves during increasing filling of the atrium of a frog heart: The "Law of the Heart" according to [1]; for further explanation see text.

Therefore, we felt the 100th anniversary of Otto Frank's publication "Zur Dynamik des Herzmuskels" not only to be a good occasion to give a review of the literature, but also to stimulate scientists due to the recent controversies regarding the existence of the FSM in failing myocardium. A consequent reevaluation of the FSM may be of great academic interest on the one hand, its clinical consequences may be of equally great importance, on the other.

In the following review, we focus on some historical aspects and report early in vivo and in vitro animal studies. Thereafter, special effort is made to dissect the specific molecular structures involved in the FSM. In the second part, potential loss or attenuation of the FSM in human congestive heart failure and the special role of myocardial distensibility in this context are critically discussed.

The fact that Otto Frank was able to discover the "Law of the Heart" already at the end of the 19th century was due to the recognition of fundamental findings in skeletal muscle physiology as well as due to the development of new methods. Fick in 1878 [10] and Blix in 1891 [13] had already demonstrated the relationship between muscle length and force development in skeletal muscle. Because Otto Frank had recognized this relationship and was aware of the fact that length and force in skeletal muscle correspond to volume and pressure of the whole heart, respectively, he started to study the relation between filling and pressure development in the whole heart for the first time. In order to be able to measure isovolumetric pressure and to control experimental conditions, he was smart enough to choose a cold-blooded heart, in particular a frog heart for reasons of metabolism and anatomical simplicity. This allowed him to cannulate the inferior vena cava thereby connecting the atrium to a manometer and a reservoir. The left ventricle was cannulated via the aorta to a second manometer, which allowed registration of ventricular pressure, and to an outflow tube, which was controlled by a stopcock allowing to select between isovolumetric and afterloaded contractions. The perfusion medium was a mixture of bovine or sheep's blood and physiologic salt solution. A typical example of his experiments is given in Figure 1: When the atrium is filled with increasing volumes (0 – 1,0 ccm) from the blood reservoir, the pressure development increased gradually in the atrium (lower diagram). According to a greater filling of the atrium, the ventricle is also filled to a greater extent, so that peak developed pressure gradually increased. Thereby, the "Law of the Heart" is demonstrated for the atrium and ventricle of the frog heart, although neither atrial nor ventricular volumes are exactly defined. This point is critically commented by Otto Frank himself: "I could proceed similarly (to plot a length-tension curve like in skeletal muscle) with respect to the heart, if I could regard maximal tensions as functions of cardiac filling. This is made difficult by the fact that in my method ventricular filling is not precisely measured." The author, Otto Frank, was aware that a "distensibility curve" (resting pressure-volume relation) is needed.

When Starling and co-workers [2] rediscovered the "Law of the Heart" some ten years later, two major differences in the experimental approach were obvious: (1) Starling and co-workers performed experiments in isolated warm-blooded hearts, and (2) they measured ventricular volumes allowing to construct pressure-volume relationships.

Despite the clear descriptions of the "Law of the Heart" in the two classic publications mentioned above, the validity and significance of this mechanism in the intact circulation of an organism have been questioned for a variety of reasons: (1) Isolated working heart preparations are artificial preparations, and do not need to reflect the true "in vivo" situation. (2) Metabolic support in isolated hearts may be inadequate. (3) Other regulation mechanisms like heart rate, sympathetic tone and other neuroendocrine systems may be superior to the Frank-Starling mechanism making the importance of the latter one less relevant.

A number of experimental animal studies have been addressed to these questions in the middle of the last century. In most of these studies the anaesthetized instrumented open- or closed-chest dog was used as a model. There is a great body of evidence from those studies that the Frank-Starling mechanism is not only present in the mammalian heart, but also plays a superior role beside other regulatory mechanisms. Representative for these experimental studies, the semantical work of Sarnoff's group is presented. In their experimental approach, pressures in the right and left atria, left ventricle and aorta were measured in addition to total aortic blood flow. Such an experimental design allows to plot left ventricular stroke volume as a function of left ventricular end-diastolic pressure. Leaving contractility of the left ventricle (LV) constant, a clear and steep rise of left ventricular stroke work was observed at low left ventricular filling pressures up to about 15 cm H_2O. Between 15 and 20 cm H_2O, the LV-function curve flattened off and ended in a plateau (Figure 2, left).

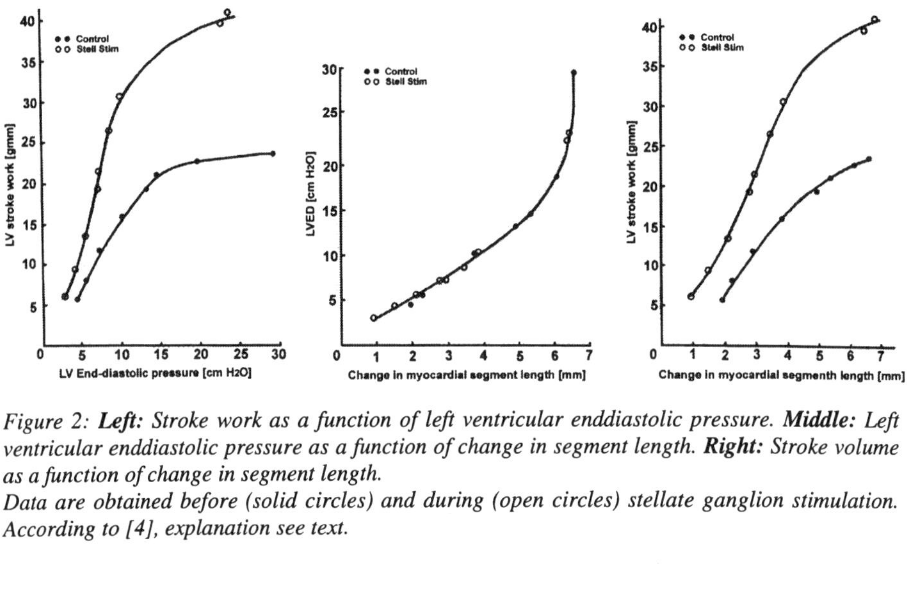

*Figure 2: **Left:** Stroke work as a function of left ventricular enddiastolic pressure. **Middle:** Left ventricular enddiastolic pressure as a function of change in segment length. **Right:** Stroke volume as a function of change in segment length.*
Data are obtained before (solid circles) and during (open circles) stellate ganglion stimulation. According to [4], explanation see text.

Interestingly, a decline of the LV function curve was never observed under standard conditions even at extremely high filling pressures. Only under conditions of myocardial ischemia, severe anemia and open pericardium, which all three may be associated with ventriculoatrial regurgitation, a decline of the LV function curve may be observed.

More important, however, is the demonstration of a family of Frank-Starling curves for each end-diastolic filling pressure. Stimulation of the sympathetic nervous system or pharmacological application of β-adrenoceptor agonists gradually shifted the LV function curve to higher stroke work values and to the left (Figure 2, left). These findings demonstrated each particular state of LV contractility to be presented by one specific Frank-Starling curve explaining the fact that stroke work may increase despite a decrease in filling pressure.

However, in these classic studies, stroke work was only related to filling pressure rather than to end-diastolic left ventricular volume as stated in the classical work of Frank and Starling. Sarnoff et al. resolved this problem by two different methodological approaches: (1) It was known from experiments in non-beating hearts [14] that the diastolic pressure-volume relationship has an exponential shape, i.e., large volume changes at lower pressures and small volume changes at higher pressures. Taking such a shape of the relationship between diastolic pressure and volume into account, the plot of stroke volume versus diastolic volume would become a more linear curve as compared to the stroke volume versus diastolic pressure relation. (2) Sarnoff et al. also experimentally analyzed segment length changes and were thereby allowed to obtain left ventricular end-diastolic pressure versus length change relations (Figure 2, middle) as well as left ventricular stroke volume versus length change relationships (Figure 2, right). This analysis not only reveals an exponential relation regarding the passive pressure-length change relationship, but also a steep and more linear left ventricular function curve (Figure 2, right). It is important to note that this analysis was performed in the dog heart with intact circulation and at constant heart rate.

The concept of the Frank-Starling mechanism can be presented in the framework of pressure-volume diagrams (Figure 3) [15].

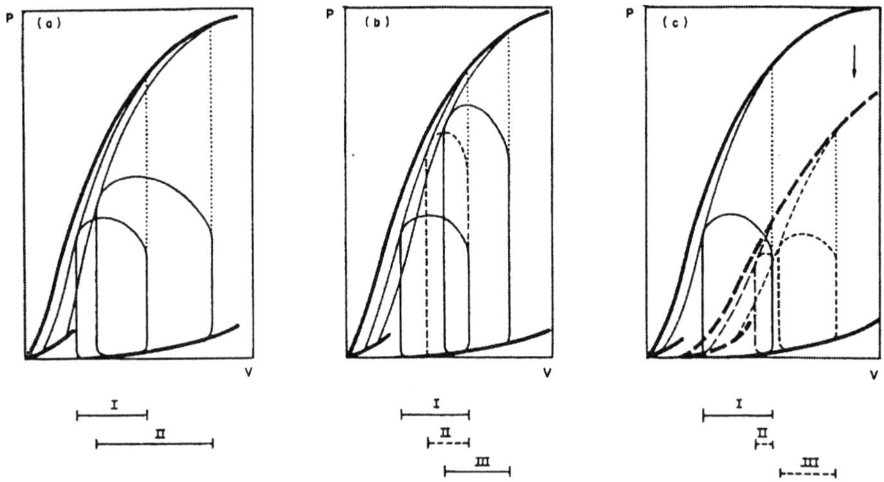

*Figure 3: **(a)** Isometric and isotonic maxima curves and pressure-volume loops at two different enddiastolic starting points. Stroke volume II is much larger than stroke volume I. **(b)** Residual volume mechansim on the basis of FSM (see text). **(c)** Compensation of loss of contractility (arrow) by FSM. Stroke volume I decreases to stroke volume II (reduction in contractility) and increases again to stroke volume III (FSM). (According to [15], see text).*

In contrast to other authors but in accordance with Otto Frank, Jacob et al. [15] demonstrate a distinction between isovolumetric maxima and the maxima of afterloaded contractions. This can be seen in Figure 3A; furthermore, two pressure volume loops for two different end-diastolic volumes are shown. The corresponding stroke volumes are given as bars at the bottom of the left diagram. As the end-diastolic volume becomes larger, the end-systolic volume does not change or increases only slightly, so that the stroke volume increases (from I to II).

Figure 3B explains the residual volume mechanism on the basis of the FSM. Elevation of aortic pressure to a high degree results in a primary decrease in stroke volume (from I to II) due to a primary increase in end-systolic volume and constant end-diastolic volume. However, as a consequence the end-diastolic volume increases and thereby a secondary rise in stroke volume (from II to III) results; in other terms, the FSM can compensate for an acute rise in aortic pressure with respect to stroke volume.

The same residual volume mechanism is present in the case of an acute decrease in LV contractility as depicted in Figure 3C. When the isovolumetric pressure-volume curve is significantly shifted downwards and to the right due to a loss of contractility, stroke volume is dramatically decreased (from I to II). This, again, may be compensated by a secondary augmentation of the end-diastolic volume thereby increasing and almost normalizing stroke volume (from II to III).

From the publications and data reported so far, it was very likely that the origin of the FSM is of cellular and molecular nature of the myocardium. Therefore, it was and still is of greatest interest to study this mechanism more directly, i.e., in multicellular skinned and non-skinned cardiac muscle preparations. Turning from whole heart experiments to isolated cardiac muscle experiments, tension or stress corresponds to pressure, and volume corresponds to muscle or sarcomere length. Although the first reports on intact isolated muscle strip preparations occurred already in 1944 and in 1954 [16,17], Sonnenblick [18] established isolated cat papillary muscle preparations in muscle physiology (see Methods: Chapter III). As shown in Figure 4, there is a clear length-dependence of peak developed isometric force, which is present in failing and non-failing mammalian myocardium [19].

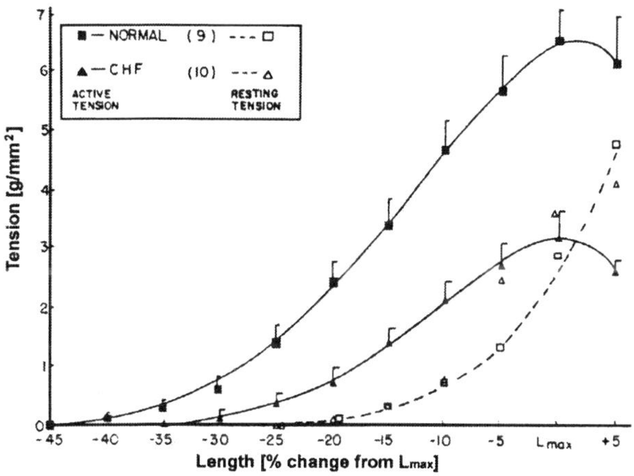

Figure 4: Length-tension relationships obtained from normal and failing cat right ventricular isolated papillary muscles according to [19]. Although active tension development is depressed in failing muscles, the FSM is still maintained.

In the past, the nature of this length-dependence of peak developed isometric force, of extent of shortening and of working capacity have been discussed by many scientists (see also Chapter III). In principle, three mechanisms may play a role in the FSM: (1) The degree of overlap of the actin and myosin filaments may correlate with the number of potentially activated cross-bridges according to the sliding filament theory as introduced by Gordon and Huxley [20]. These authors found four different relationships between developed force and sarcomere length in tetanized skeletal muscle (Figure 5).

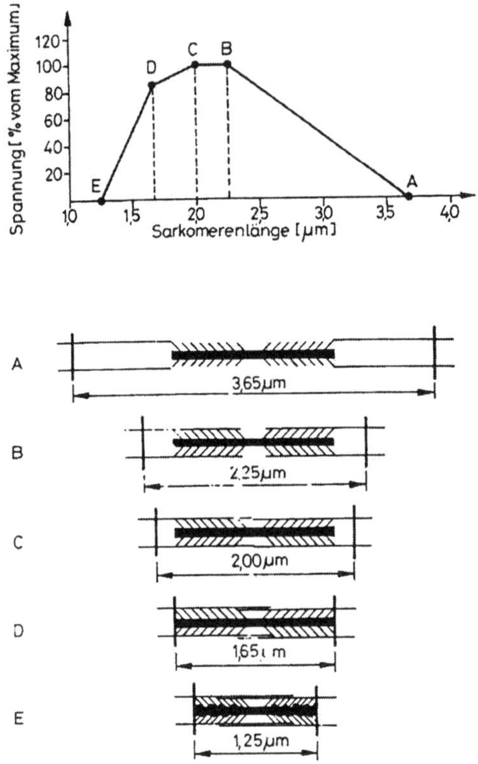

Figure 5: Relationship between force development ***(upper panel)*** *and sarcomere length* ***(lower panels A-E)*** *according to [20].*

In the length range A-B (sarcomere length between 2.25 and 3.6 µm) the degree of overlap increases gradually with decreasing sarcomere length. Between B and C, there is an ideal overlap (sarcomere length 2.0 - 2.25 µm) resulting in maximum force development, because all cross-bridges can be recruited by activation. Further reduction of sarcomere length reduces the number of available cross-bridges (range C-D and range D-E). (2) The second explanation for the nature of the FSM would be a length-dependence on activation, i.e., the number of calcium ions released from the sarcoplasmic reticulum may be larger at long than at short muscle length [21]. However, experiments with aequorin-loaded cardiac muscle preparations revealed that rapid changes in muscle length do not or only minimally influence calcium transients (Figure 6) [22].

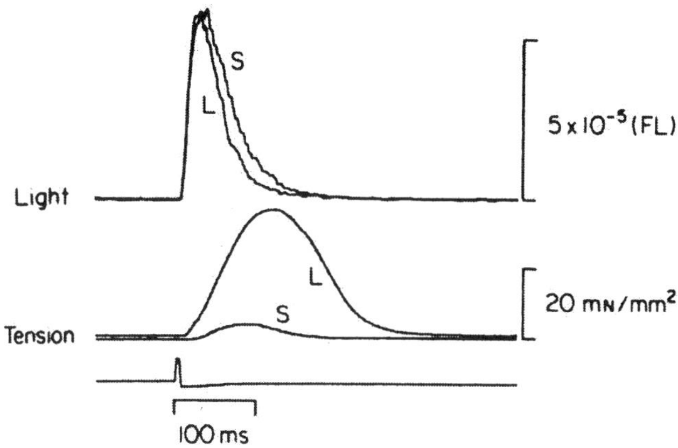

Figure 6: Tension development and calcium transients (light) in isolated cardiac muscle according to [22]. A rapid increase in length (from S to L) increases tension but without changes in the aequorin light signal (see text).

However, slow changes in developed force following muscle length changes may well be attributed to calcium transient alterations. The question whether slow changes in calcium transients are due to an increase in sarcoplasmic reticulum loading or due to an increase in the calcium inward current is not answered yet. (3) Compared to the mentioned mechanisms (1) and (2), the third mechanism is the most important one and might easily explain the greatest part of the FSM: Sarcomere length-dependent sensitivity of the regulatory proteins for calcium. This principle is shown in Figure 7 based on skinned fiber experiments performed by Kentish et al. [23].

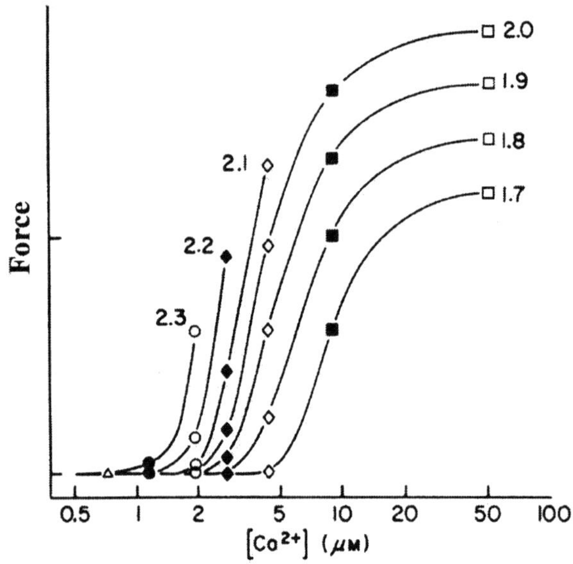

Figure 7: Relationship between [Ca^{2+}] and force development is sarcomere length dependent: Increase in force and leftward shift of the activation curve with increasing sarcomere length. Skinned fiber experiments according to [23].

These experiments show a leftward shift of the activation curves with increasing sarcomere length (Figure 7) indicating that there is no tension development at a sarcomere length of 1.7 μm but almost maximum tension development at sarcomere lengths above 2.0 μm at a Ca^{2+}-concentration of, for example, 5 μM.

Quite recently, an attenuation or even a loss of the FSM has been reported in the literature [11,12]. Therefore, we have reinvestigated the FSM in the human failing and non-failing heart on the organ, tissue and sarcomere levels. Figure 8 shows a pressure-volume relationship measured in isolated failing (n=5) and non-failing (n=2) human hearts.

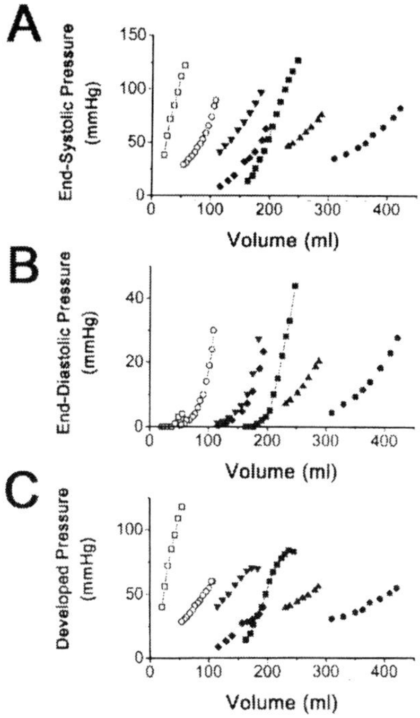

*Figure 8: **A:** Pressure-volume relationships in 2 normal (white symbols) and 5 failing human, isolated left ventricles (black symbols). **B:** Diastolic pressure-volume relationships of the same human ventricles. **C:** Developed pressure versus volume in 2 normal and 5 failing left human ventricles. According to [24].*

In comparison to the normal hearts, all pressure-volume relationships are shifted towards larger volumes in the failing hearts. Therefore, maximum ventricular performance is reached at much higher volumes compared with normal ventricles [24]. Furthermore, length-tension diagrams as well as resting tension-active tension diagrams were analyzed from experiments performed in isolated muscle strip preparations obtained from failing and non-failing left ventricles (Figure 9).

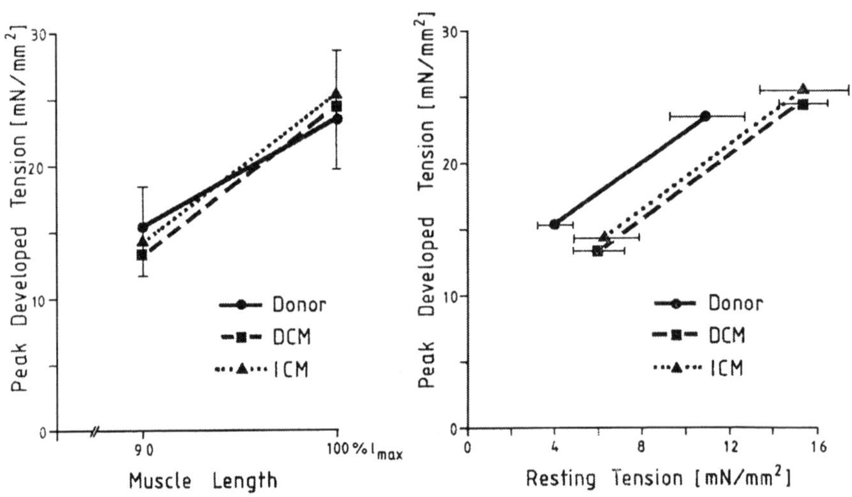

Figure 9: ***Left:*** *Length-tension relationship obtained from left ventricular muscle strip preparations from normal hearts (Donor) and failing hearts (DCM, dilated cardiomyopathy; ICM, ischemic cardiomyopathy). There is no evidence for an attenuation of the FSM.* ***Right:*** *Resting tension vs. peak developed tension relationship from the same muscle preparation as in the left diagram. Resting tension is higher in DCM and ICM as compared to normal, whereas peak developed tension is similiar in all three experimental groups.* According to [24].

There is clear evidence that within the physiological range (90 % to 100 % L_{max} (optimal length)) there is an increase in peak developed force by about 70 % both in failing and non-failing myocardium [24]. In order to demonstrate that the length-dependence of Ca^{2+}-sensitivity is also present in these failing hearts, skinned fibers were exposed to different Ca^{2+}-concentrations at two different sarcomere lengths (1.9 and 2.3 µm) as measured by laser diffraction. Again, like in normal mammalian fibers, an increase in sarcomere length results in an leftward shift of the force-pCa curve (Figure 10) [24].

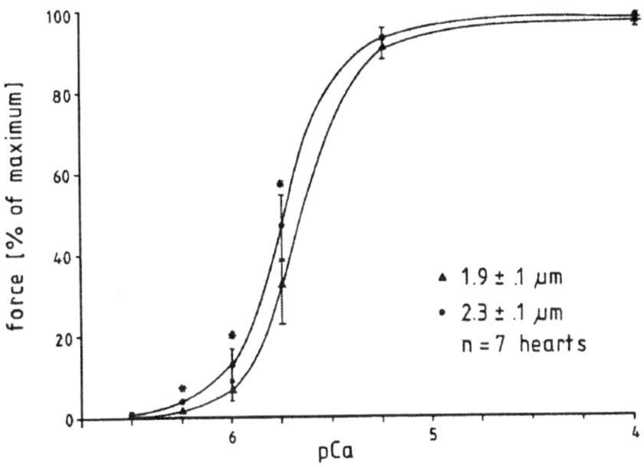

Figure 10: pCa-force relationship at two different sarcomere lengths (1.9µm and 2.3µm) obtained from human left ventricular skinned fibers. The activation curve is significantly shifted to the left with increasing sarcomere length, the major mechanism of the FSM.
According to [24].

These data, taken together, provide clear evidence that the FSM is indeed present in human myocardium and is not essentially changed in the failing hearts. The importance of the FSM in the vivo situation lies mainly in the adaptation of the left to the right ventricular stroke volume. However, the FSM is also essential for increases in stroke volume under conditions of physiological exercise.

REFERENCES

1) Frank O: Zur Dynamik des Herzmuskels. J Biol 1895;32:370-447. Translation from German: Chapman CP, Wasserman EB. Am Heart J 1959;58:282-317

2) Starling EH: Linacre lecture on the law of the heart. Longmans, London 1918

3) Bowditch HP: Ueber die Eigentuemlichkeiten der Reizbarkeit welche Muskelfasern des Herzen zeigen. Ber Sachs Ges Akkad 1871;23:652-689

4) Sarnoff SJ, Brodman SK, Gilmore JP, Linden RJ, Mitchell JH: Regulation of ventricular contraction, influence of cardiac sympathetic and vagal nerve stimulation on atrial and ventricular dynamics. Circ Res 1960;8;1108-1122

5) Koch-Weser J: Myocardial action of angiotensin. Circ Res 1964;14:337-343

6) Holubarsch Ch, Hasenfuss G, Schmidt-Schweda S, Knorr A, Pieske B, Ruf T, Fasol R, Just H: Angiotensin I and II exert inotropic effects in atrial but not in ventricular human myocardium. Circulation 1993;88:1228-1237

7) Krämer BK, Smith TW, Kelly RA: Endothelin and increased contractility in adult rat ventricular myocytes. Circ Res 1991;68:269-279

8) Holubarsch C, Pieske B, Kretschmann B, Schmidt-Schweda S, Meyer M, Schlotthauer K, Ruf T, Hasenfuss G, Just H: The functional role of angiotensin and endothelin in failing and non-failing human myocardium. In: Dhalla NS, Beanish RE, Takeda N, Nagano M, eds. The Failing Heart. Philadelphia, Pa: Lippincot-Raven Publishers 1995:295-304

9) Kelly RA, Eid H, Krüger BK, et al: Endothelin enhances the contractile responsiveness of adult rat ventricular myocytes to calcium by a pertussis toxin-sensitive pathway. J Clin Invest 1990;86:1164-1171

10) Fick A: Über die Wärmeentwicklung bei der Muskelzuckung. Pflügers Arch Physiol 1878;16;59-90

11) Böhm M, Beuckelmann KDJ, Schwinger RHG, Erdmann E: Aktuelle pathophysiologische Aspekte der Herzinsuffizienz. Internist 1003;34:886-901

12) Schwinger RHG, Böhm M, Koch A, Schmidt U, Morano J, Eissner H-J, Überfuhr R, Reichart B, Erdmann E: The failing heart is unable to use the Frank-Starling mechanism. Circ Res 1994;74:959-90

13) Blix, M: Die Länge und Spannung des Muskels. Skandinav Arch Physiol Leipzig 1891;3:295-318

14) Isaacs JP, Carter BN, Haller JA: Experimental pericarditis: The pathologic physiology of constrictive pericarditis. Bull. Johns Hopkins Hosp 1952;90:259

15) Jacob R, Dierberger B, Kissling G: Functional significance of the Frank-Starling mechanism under physiological and pathophysiological conditions. Eur Heart J 1992;13:Suppl E 7-14

16) Lundin G: Mechanical properties of cardiac muscle. Acta Physiol Scand 1944;7:Supp 20

17) Abbot BC, Mommaerts WFHM: A study of inotropic mechanisms in the papillary muscle preparation. J Gen Physiol 1959;42:533-551

18) Sonnenblick EH: Force-velocity relations in mammalian heart muscle. Am J Physiol 1962;202:931-939

19) Spann JF, Covell JW, Eckberg KL, Sonnenblick EH, Ross J, Braunwald E: Contractile performance of the hypertrophied and chronically failing cat ventricle. Am J Physiol 1972;223:1150-1157

20) Gordon AM, Huxley AF, Julian FJ: The variation in isometric tension with sarcomere length in vertebrate muscle fibre. J Physiol 1966;184:170-192

21) Fabiato A, Fabiato F: Dependence of the contractile activation of skinned cardiac cells on the sarcomere length. Nature 1975;256:54-56

22) Allen DG, Kentish JC: The cellular basis of the length-tension relation in cardiac muscle. J Mol Cell Cardiol 1985;17:821-840

23) Kentish JC, TerKeurs HEDJ, Noble MIM, Riccardi L, Schouten VJA: The relationships between force, [Ca2+] and sarcomere length in skinned trabeculae from rat ventricle. J Physiol 1983;345:24P

24) Holubarsch Ch, Ruf T, Goldstein DJ, Ashton RC, Nickl W, Pieske B, Pioch K, Lüdemann J, Wiesner S, Hasenfuss G, Posival H, Just H, Burkhoff D: Existence of the Frank-Starling mechanism in the failing human heart. Investigations on the organ, tissue, and sacromere length. Circulation 1996; 94: 683-689

II. THE MYOTHERMAL METHOD: HISTORICAL AND PERSONAL ASPECTS

In 1976, I met Norman R. Alpert for the first time on occasion of a symposium held at the University of Tübingen, Germany, and organized by my former mentor Prof. Dr. Ruthard Jacob, Chairmen of Physiology, University of Tübingen. After I had just finished my thesis of medicine entitled "Force-velocity relations in the cat papillary muscle", I had the chance to listen to my first lesson on cardiac energetics: "The Partitioning of Altered Mechanics in Hypertrophied Heart Muscle between the Sarcoplasmic Reticulum and the Contractile Apparatus by Means of Myothermal Measurements", which later has been published by N.R. Alpert and L.A. Mulieri [1]. This was the first time that I was attracted by this specific method to study cardiac muscle function and energetics. Only two years later I studied the phenomenon of hypoxic and glucose deficiency contracture in rat cardiac muscle at the Department of Physiology Tübingen, Germany (Figure 1 [2]).

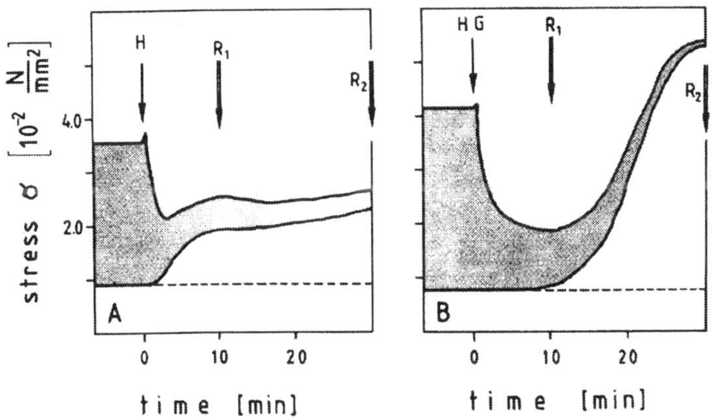

Figure 1: Isometric force development of rat left ventricular papillary muscle preparation. ***A:*** *Response to hypoxia (H; $pO_2 < 10$ mmHg): Developed force immediately decreases and diastolic force gradually increases.* ***B:*** *Response to oxygen and glucose deficiency (HG): Developed force decreases and diastolic force increases to stress values even higher than peak developed force of twitch at control conditions. R_1 and R_2 indicate at which timepoints reversibility tests were performed. According to [2].*

Immediately, I knew that a myothermal analysis of this phenomenon could be an ideal approach for better understanding of the fundamental mechanisms involved in diastolic contracture.

Therefore, I applied for a travelling grant for a scientific stay at the University of Vermont/Burlington/USA in N.R. Alpert's laboratory. I was happy to receive this grant from the Dr. Erwin-Riesch-Foundation of the University Tübingen in 1979. To get prepared in an optimal way prior to my departure from Germany, I very carefully studied the literature of skeletal [3] and cardiac [4] muscle energetics. I was especially interested in the bibliography of A.V. Hill entitled "Trails and Trials in Physiology" [3]. When reading the introduction to this book of A.V. Hill, I learnt to know that this scientist had been working in the same Department of Physiology, probably even in the same lab, at the University of Tübingen, in which I studied muscle mechanics for at least five years. Interestingly, A.V. Hill started in this institution his career in muscle energetics in 1911. He was attracted by a paper of Bürker who was at that time Professor of Physiology in Tübingen. This paper was published in 1908 with the title "Methoden zur Thermodynamik des Muskels" [5]. This paper and the myothermal method already available at this time led A.V. Hill to Tübingen. He wrote about his stay in Tübingen: "His 1908 paper (Bürker's paper) led me in 1911 to spend two months with him (Prof. Bürker) in the pleasant little university town of Tübingen"[3].

I myself lived for almost thirty years in Tübingen including school education, study of medicine, and habilitation (Ph. D.) for Physiology. A.V. Hill wrote further: "There I learnt about his (Bürker's) methods of constructing thermopiles and had the great good fortune to meet Friedrich Paschen, the Professor of Physics and a famous contributor to infrared spectroscopy. Later, from 1924 on, Paschen was Director of the Physikalisch-Technische Reichsanstalt in Berlin until he was dismissed by the Nazis in 1933 and replaced by the notorious Johannes Stark; in 1928 he was Rumford medallist of the Royal Society. With characteristic good nature, and often with loud shouts of laughter, Paschen taught me about his fine moving-magnet galvanometers, and he allowed me to carry away in my bag (for 80 marks) a beautiful iron-shielded instrument made in his laboratory. This galvanometer lived three and a half years in my cellar, among cages of Hopkin's rats, and in 1914 was used by Weizsäcker and Parnas to make their experiments, too. Paschen's generous advice was available again, from 1920, when we started constructing galvanometers like his in England. Bürker later published another paper on methods, but it contained little new. The kindly help of Bürker and Paschen in 1911 gave a start to the improvements of technique which have continued since for many years, largely at other people's hands: Weizsäcker's in 1914, Fenn's in 1922, Hartree's from

1919 to 1933, and Downing's from 1920 to the present day. But that is another story which will be told later."

Before I will come back to my own experiences with muscle mechanics and energetics using also the myothermal method, I would like to mention the scientific contribution of Viktor Weizsäcker. He went a very similar scientific way as I did exactly 65 years later. Weizsäcker, at that time at Heidelberg, had been occupied with the comparison of mechanical work and oxygen consumption in frogs' hearts and also with the inhibiting effects of cyanide. At 1914, Weizsäcker went to Cambridge to A.V. Hill's laboratory: He found out that the so-called initial heat, which is immediately released during the muscle contraction, was independent of the presence of oxygen and unaltered by application of cyanide. From his findings it could be concluded that the chemical reactions that release the energy for the primary process of contraction are independent of oxygen [6]. This finding was the basis of our understanding of muscle energetics: ATP, the providing molecule for energy, is present in muscle to a great amount. This molecule is split during the contraction process and energy is liberated which can be measured as work and/or initial heat. Thereafter, ATP is resynthesized using energy from the reaction of substrates and oxygen. The heat liberated during this latter reaction is called recovery heat, and the process itself is named recovery process. A.V. Hill wrote about the stay of v. Weizsäcker in Cambridge: "However, his final contribution to it (physiology) was a fundamental one; its merit lays in asking (in Heidelberg) the right question and then going where the technique was available." Later on v. Weizsäcker abandoned physiology and was more interested in clinical neurology. In 1941, he was appointed to the Chair of Neurology at Breslau.

When I was reading Weizsäcker's scientific history in 1979, I was quite astonished about the parallels between his and my situation. I had been working on the mechanisms of hypoxic contracture (see Figure 1). The main question, which immediately came up, was whether the diastolic "contracture" tension is active, i.e., maintained by calcium-activated cross-bridges thereby consuming energy, or is passive, i.e., generated by rigor cross-bridges thereby consuming no or very little energy. It seemed to me that the myothermal approach would be the most straightforward method to answer this question. Therefore, I decided to go and to study where the method is available: Burlington/Vermont/USA. At that time, L.A. Mulieri and N.R. Alpert had just successfully constructed a new thermopile which was improved a lot (1) by using antimony and bismuth as metals and (2) by changing from handmade thermopiles to vacuum-deposition of the metals onto the mica sheets [7].

When I arrived in October 1979 in the wonderful landscape of Vermont, I was immediately allowed to work with these newly developed thermopiles, and only a few months later, we were able to answer the question of the nature of hypoxic contracture. Figure 2 shows the decisive analysis of our data obtained in rat left ventricular trabeculae.

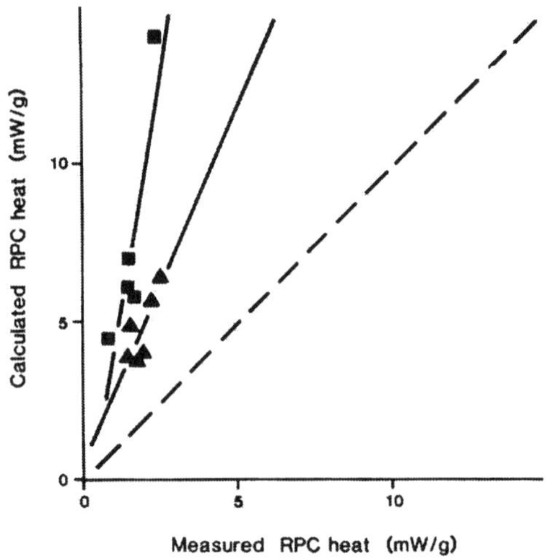

Figure 2: Relationship between measured RPC heat and calculated RPC heat for KCl contracture (---), hypoxic contracture (-▲-), and oxygen and glucose deficiency contracture (-■-). RPC, resting heat plus contracture heat. RPC heat is much lower in contractures due to hypoxia or deficiency of oxygen and glucose as compared to KCl contracture. According to [8].

Compared to a potassium chloride induced contracture, there was no evidence that hypoxic contracture is associated with a relevant release of energy indicating that oxygen and/or glucose deficiency contracture is mainly due to rigor bonds between actin and myosin [8].

Stimulated by these data which were published in Circulation Research [8], I continued to study muscle energetics for the next several years (up to now) by organizing several scientific stays at the University of Vermont. The cooperation and friendship with L.A. Mulieri and N.R. Alpert were the basis for many years of very fruitful and successful scientific work (see chapter IV).

REFERENCES

1) Alpert NR, Mulieri LA: The partitioning of altered mechanics in hypertrophied heart muscle between the sarcoplasmic reticulum and the contractile apparatus by means of myothermal measurement. Basic Res Cardiol 1977;72:153-159

2) Holubarsch Ch, Jacob R: Diastolic tension of rat cardiac muscle during deficiency of oxygen and glucose. Stress-strain relationships and reversibilitiy. Basic Res Cardiol 1981;76:690-703

3) Hill AV: Trails and trials in physiology. A Bibliography. Edward Arnold (Publishers) LTD London 1960

4) Gibbs C: Cardiac energetics. Physiol Rev 1978;58:174-254

5) Bürker K: Handb. (Tigerstedt) physiol. Meth. 1908;2:1-86

6) Weizsäcker V: Initial heat is independent of presence of oxygen. J Physiol 1914;48:396-427

7) Mulieri LA, Luhr G, Trefry J, Alpert NR: Metal-film thermopiles for use with rabbit right ventricular papillary muscles. Am J Physiol 1977;233:C146-156

8) Holubarsch Ch, Alpert NR, Goulette R, Mulieri LA: Heat production during hypoxic contracture of rat myocardium. Circ Res 1982;51:777-786

3. PAPILLARY MUSCLE EXPERIMENTS

3.1. Introduction

Before the sixties of the last century, performance of the heart has been described exclusively on the basis of data from the whole heart either in vivo or in an isolated fashion. In contrast to muscle physiology performed in isolated skeletal muscle, however, those studies did not allow to draw final conclusions on myocardial contraction per se, because of (1) the special geometry and complex architecture of the heart as a whole, and because of (2) the complex reflex situation of the heart when studied within the integrated circulation. Therefore, isolated longitudinally orientated cardiac muscle preparations were very promising to elucidate clearly the specific effects of preload and afterload (mechanical conditions), the influence of heart rate as well as of neuroendocrine mechanisms, as there are catecholamines, angiotensins, endothelins and others. The basic physical parameters of myocardial contraction are described by (1) a length-tension diagram on the one hand (Figure 1) and (2) a force-velocity diagram on the other hand (Figure 2).

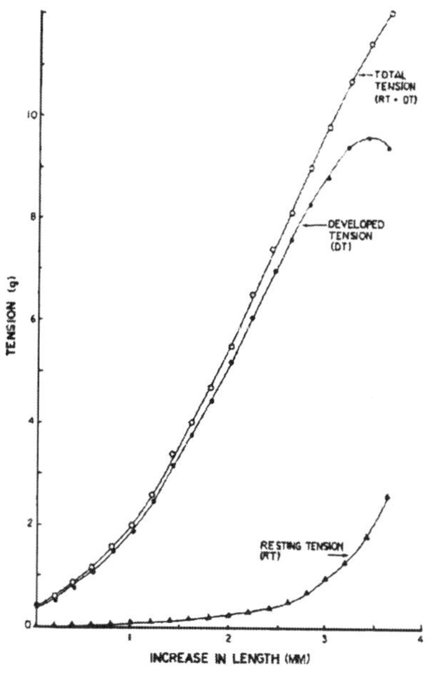

Figure 1: Length-tension diagram of a cat papillary muscle. Initial length 12 mm. Experimental temperature 22°C. Stimulation rate 30/min. According to [6].

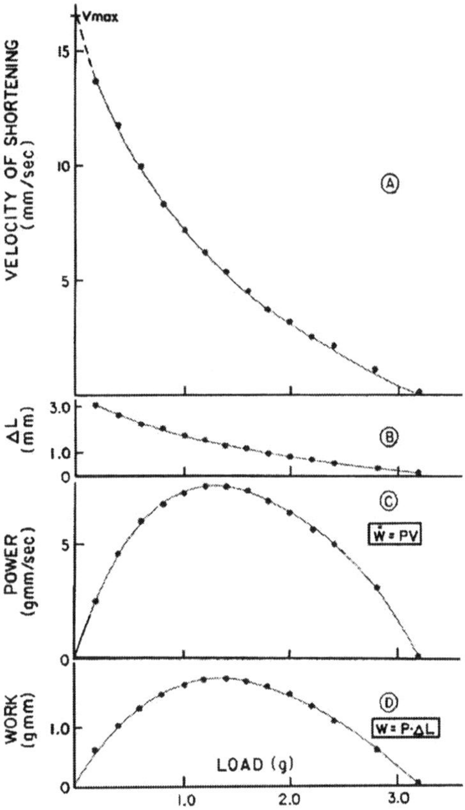

*Figure 2: **A.** Force-velocity relation. **B.** Extent of shortening as a function of load. **C.** Power output as a function of load. **D.** Work output as a function of load.*
Data obtained from a cat papillary muscle. Initial muscle length 12 mm, experimental temperature 21°C, stimulation rate 30/min. According to [6].

Furthermore, there are not only physiological needs and questions which may be resolved by such a longitudinal preparation similar to a skeletal muscle; pathophysiological (failing myocardium) as well as pharmacological studies have followed quickly after establishing this elegant method of isolated papillary or trabecular muscle preparation. Whereas in the sixties and seventies those experiments with isolated cardiac muscle tissues were restricted to animal tissues (rat, cat, rabbit, guinea pig, dog), later on, due to the increasing number of heart transplantations worldwide, human cardiac tissue became available for studying muscle mechanics in failing and non-failing preparations. It should also be emphasized that isolated cardiac muscle preparations play a great role in search for new cardiovascular compounds, especially positive inotropic ones, but also for toxicological tests for new compounds with other than cardiovascular indications.

3.2. Methods

Regarding studies with isolated longitudinal cardiac muscle preparations several methodological aspects must be considered: (1) Bathing solutions, (2) the size of the preparation (thickness, length), (3) the instruments and procedures used for muscle preparation, (4) the types of fixation of both ends of the muscle, (5) electrical stimulation, (6) the mechanical apparatus allowing only isometric or isometric and isotonic and even auxotonic contractions, and (7) the study protocol regarding mounting the muscle and stretching procedures.

Ad (1): Regarding the composition of bathing solutions, a variety of solutions have been used in the past and are used at present. In this article, we would like to focus only on calcium concentrations and the use of BDM (butanedione-monoxime). In the first experiments with isolated cardiac muscles, calcium concentrations were chosen to be high, i.e., between 2.5 and 5.6 mM. In the standard Krebs-Ringer solution, which we used during most of our studies in the last 20 years, calcium concentration was 2.5 mM. However, it might be that even 2.5 mM calcium concentration is too high for the following two reasons: (1) In the human serum, calcium concentration is around 2.5 mM; however, half of it is certainly bound to proteins so that the free calcium concentration may be about 1.25 mM. (2) Especially in rat myocardium, force of contraction is maximum already at a calcium concentration of 2.5 mM. Therefore, influences of physiological or pharmacological interventions on myocardial force might be detectable only at lower calcium concentrations (own observations). Since about 1988, many scientists use BDM added to the bathing solution during transportation and preparation for the following reasons: BDM provides protection of the myocardium (1) by blocking the actin-myosin interaction (desensitization for calcium ions) and thereby preventing contracture (permanent diastolic calcium dependent tone), and (2) by blocking the calcium channels and ameloriating calcium overload. Most importantly, these blocking effects are quickly and completely reversible [1,2,3].

Ad (2): In the pioneer experiments, preparations were used with relatively large sizes regarding especially muscle diameter or cross-sectional area. However, rapidly it became clear that muscle preparations thicker than 1.0

mm diameter (= 0.8 mm^2 cross-sectional area) tended to deteriorate with time depending on experimental temperature and the study protocol (heart rate, catecholamines, etc.).

Later on, when human tissues were used and experimental temperature was chosen to be physiological, i.e., 37 °C, even lower cross-sectional areas were needed. In order to guarantee adequate oxygenation throughout the whole muscle strip, the Paradise test [4] was often used in our laboratory: The stability of the preparation, i.e., the constancy of isometric force development, was tested during continuous reduction of the oxygen partial pressure. It was shown that cross-sectional areas of less than 0.6 mm^2 are acceptable for those experiments [6].

Because any method used to fix both ends of the muscle preparation to the apparatus (see below) must induce some damage to the muscle tissue, muscle preparations are to be chosen as long as possible minimizing the effect of damaged ends on internal shortening and thereby on measured force and velocity parameters.

Ad (3): When scientific investigations in isolated papillary muscles were started, papillary muscles were removed from the right ventricle simply by cutting the upper tendon and the lower muscular basis as quick as possible using only the naked eye. Later on, especially when smaller preparations had to be cut out of large papillary muscles or the free wall of human left ventricles, care was taken for careful visualization of cardiac muscle structures (fibrosis, fiber orientation) by the use of a microscope (for example VMT Olympus). Furthermore, these cutting procedures were performed in specially designed dissection chambers and by the help of micro-dissection scissors and finest forceps.

Ad (4): As already mentioned, the damage induced by the fixation method may play a critical role. There are at least three principal methods described and used in order to guarantee perfect contact between the vital muscle tissue and the apparatus (see Figure 3):

(1) A number of scientists have clamped the muscles by the use of metal clips on each end. The advantage of using this method is twofold: The procedure is relatively simply and the connection is strong, i.e., without extra compliance. The disadvantage results clearly from the mechanical damage due to clamping the cylindrical muscles (Figure 3B).
(2) Over the years, in our lab we used a combination of a small steel hook and a silk ligature. This combination was used, because we thought that very little damage is induced by the use of the steel hook. Because a thin steel hook alone may change its position within the muscle during contraction and

stretching procedures, its position needs to be secured by an additional ligature (Figure 3A).

(3) Especially in myothermal experiments, when metal cannot be used because of its heat capacity, only silk loops and silk ligatures can be applied (Figure 3C). The disadvantage necessarily resides in the extra compliance inherent to the system.

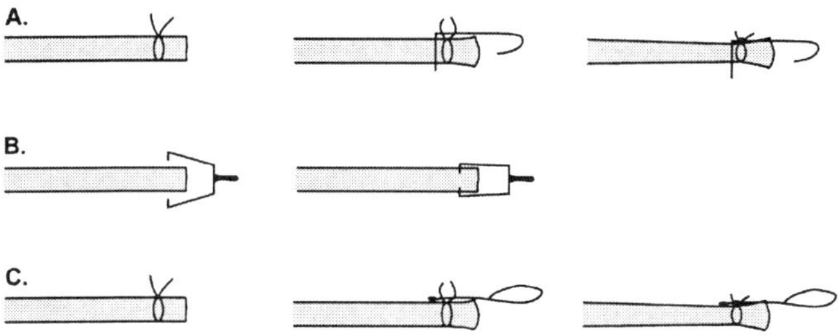

Figure 3: Three different methods to fix a muscle preparation in a muscle bath. ***A.*** *Use of hooks and ligatures.* ***B.*** *Use of steel-clampes.* ***C.*** *Use of silk ligatures only.*

Ad (5): In most of the experiments performed and the apparatus used, field stimulation is used provided by two platinum plates on both sides of the muscle. Again, for myothermal experiments metal material has to be avoided. Therefore, two very thin platinum wires (20 μm) are integrated into two silk loops at both ends of the muscle providing an end-to-end stimulation. Usually, stimulation duration is chosen to be 5 msec, and the voltage is set to be 25 % above threshold. The voltage necessary to stimulate the muscle depends on the stimulation design (see above) and the quality of preparation.

Ad (6): When only isometric experiments are to be performed, the mechanical apparatus is quite simple. One end of the muscle (loops, clips, hooks) is connected to a fixed hook or stylus the position of which is controlled by a micrometer screw providing a diastolic lengthening and shortening, i.e., stretching and destretching of the muscle. The other end of the muscle (loops, clips, hooks) is connected to a force transducer. In principle, force has been measured by three types of force transducers in the past: the electromagnetic force transducer, the capacitance-type force transducer, and the piezo-electrical force transducer. Especially, when fast processes are to be measured, only the latter one may be used because of its high resonance frequency. The apparatus becomes much more sophisticated, when afterloaded contractions are to be allowed providing measurements of velocity and constructions of force-velocity curves and length-tension loops. For these purposes, one end of the muscle must be connected to a force transducer (see above) and the other to an isotonic lever. In former days, the position of the lever was controlled by an electromagnetic coil and a stop screw (see Figure 4).

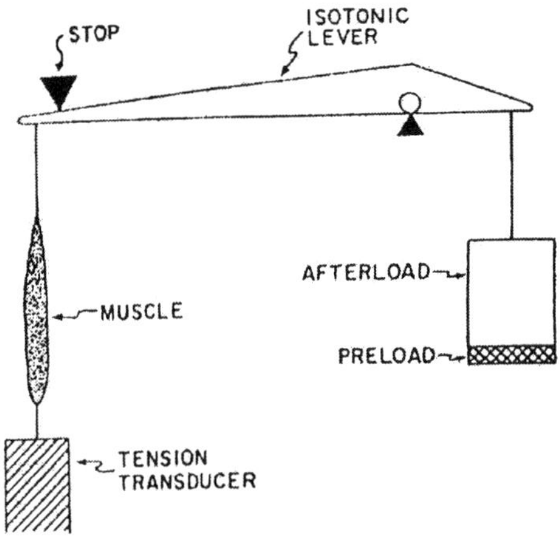

Figure 4: Experimental setup for performing afterloaded contractions: By using a stop-screw the position of the isotonic lever and thereby the preload can be controlled. [According to 6].

The current delivered to the coil was then proportional to the preload (without stop screw established) and to the afterload (with stop screw established as preload control) [6].

Modern systems, which are commercially available (for example, Muscle Research System, Scientific Instruments, Heidelberg, Germany), make use of a linear motor controlled by an electronic servo-unit allowing programmed muscle contractions.

Ad (7): Everything has to be done to prevent damage to the muscle preparation. The idea which led to the application of BDM during the transportation and preparation_procedure has been discussed. More importantly is the prevention of mechanical damage to the muscle: Care must be taken to avoid uncontrolled stretch of the muscle during preparation procedure (ligatures, cutting, loops, hooks) and during mounting the muscle. Mounting the muscle in the apparatus should be performed without any mechanical stretch, i.e., initial stretching of the muscle should not result in any diastolic force. In some study protocols, a minimum initial force of 2.5 mN preload has been accepted. In this unstretched position, the muscle should be left for quite a while (between 30 min to 1 h). During this period of time, BDM is to be washed out eventually, and electrical stimulation should be started. After this recovery and equilibration period, the muscle should be stretched by 0.05 mm or 0.1 mm increases in muscle length allowing enough time for relaxation between the steps. Stretching procedure before reaching l_{max}, the optimum length, at which maximum peak developed tension is reached, may last up to one hour. Thereafter, another relaxation and recovery period of 30 min to 1 h is recommended before the specific study protocol may be started.

3.3. Results

3.3.1. Isometric Experiments

3.3.1.1. Animal Studies: Acute Interventions

In order to construct length-tension diagrams, longitudinal muscle preparations might be stepwise stretched from l_0, the muscle length at which diastolic, passive tension is virtually zero, to l_{max}, the muscle length at which systolic, active tension is maximum (see Figure 5).

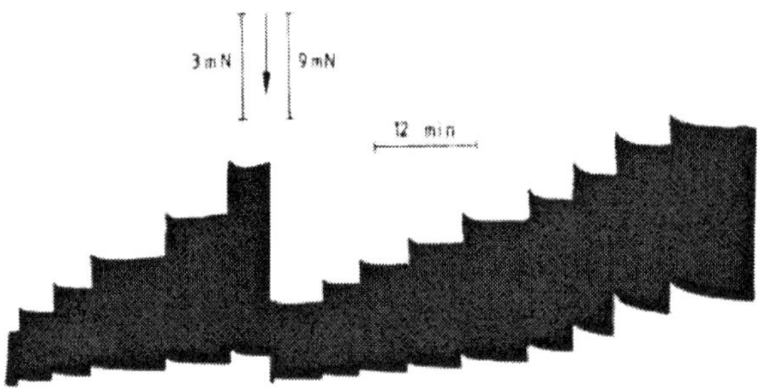

Figure 5: Original record of stretching procedure of a human muscle preparation. Muscle is stretched using 0.05 mm steps. Muscle length at l_{max} was 5.4 mm; crossectional area 0.46 mm^2. Arrow indicates change in amplification. Note the duration of stretching procedure.

Plotting the diastolic and peak systolic tension values as a function of the respective muscle length, the typical isometric length-tension diagrams are obtained (Figure 6).

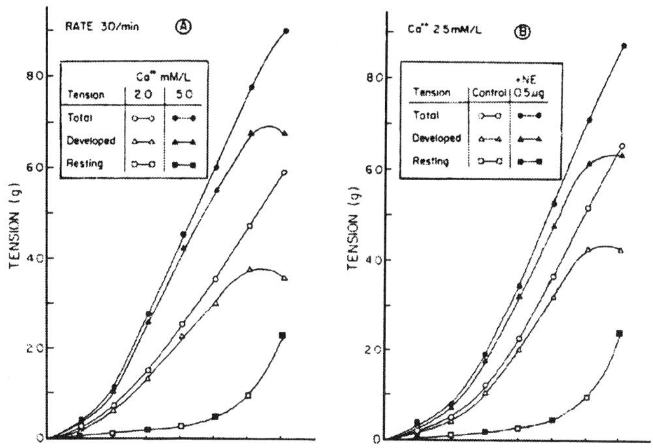

*Figure 6: Influence of 5.0 mM calcium (**A**) and 0.5 µg norepinephrine (**B**) on length-tension relation. According to [7].*

These diagrams represent the basis of the so-called Frank-Starling mechanism (Chapter I). Positive inotropic interventions like high calcium, isoproterenol, digoxin, phosphodiesterase inhibitors and calcium sensitizers acutely increase peak developed tension over the whole physiological range of muscle length (Figure 6) [7]. Bowditch has shown the dependence of the strength of the heart beat on the stimulation frequency about 100 years ago [8]. This observation has been proven in isolated muscle preparations [6]. In Figure 7, a typical own experiment (a papillary muscle) is shown. A positive force-frequency relationship is demonstrated.

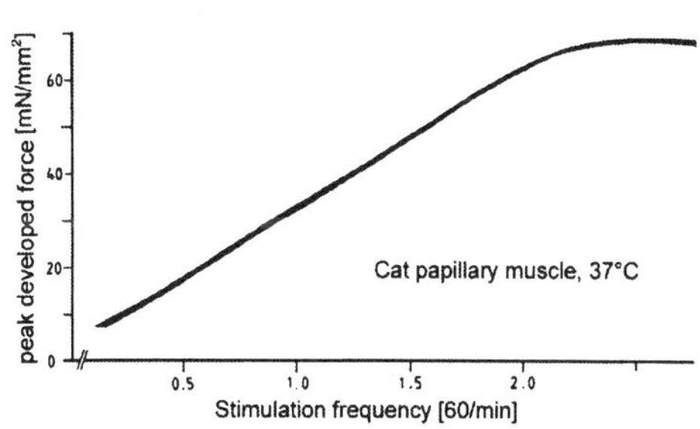

Figure 7: Force-frequency relationship in a cat papillary muscle at 37°C. With increasing frequencies developed force is also enhanced.

Furthermore, already very early, positive inotropic actions of angiotensin II have been demonstrated in cat papillary muscles [9]. Own experiments show concentration-dependent positive inotropic effects of angiotensin II in left ventricular preparations of hamsters (Figure 8) [10].

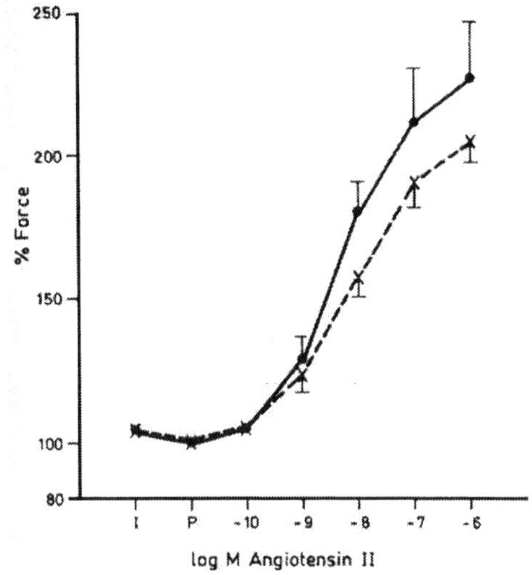

Figure 8: Dose-response curves for angiotensin II in left ventricular preparations of hamsters. Hamster myocardium responded to angiotensin II (10^{-6} M) with an increase in peak developed tension from 100% to 226%±19%. Use of BDM-containing solution for protection during transportation and preparation over 6 hours
(x---x) had no significant effect compared to immediately performed experiments without BDM (•—•). According to [10]

3.1.2. Animal Studies: Chronic Alterations

Chronic diseases like cardiac hypertrophy induced by arterial hypertension or right heart failure induced by pulmonary constriction may differently influence the length-tension diagram of the myocardium obtained from animals studied in specific models: (1) Spann et al. [11] investigated right ventricular muscles of failing hearts due to pulmonary constriction (Figure 9).

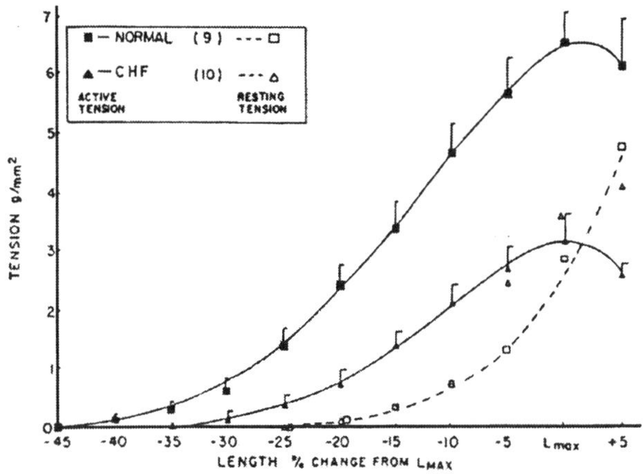

Figure 9: Length-tension diagram from normal and failing cat right ventricular isolated papillary muscles according to [11]. Active (developed) tension is depressed, but length-dependency of force development is maintained.

Systolic peak force development was depressed. (2) We found an increase in systolic peak developed force in Golblatt rats (renal hypertension) and in SHR rats (spontaneous hypertension) [12]. However, in later stages of the disease, peak developed force decreased to about 50 % of normal [13].

3.1.3. Human Studies: Acute and Chronic Interventions

A typical length-tension curve of a failing human muscle preparation (DCM, NYHA IV) is shown in Figure 10 [14].

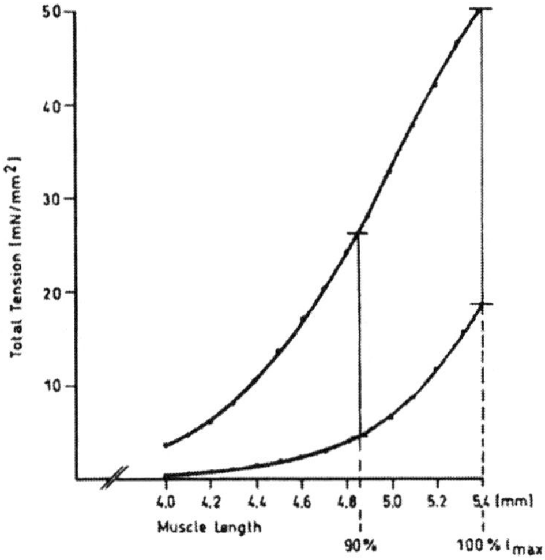

Figure 10: Typical length-tension curve of a failing human muscle preparation obtained from the left ventricle (DCM, NYHA IV). Length-dependency of force development is obviously present.

The Frank-Starling mechanism is obviously preserved in this experiment (for further discussion see Chapter I).

For many years, downregulation of β-adrenoceptors and therefore reduced response to β-adrenoceptor stimulation have been known (Figure 11) in failing human myocardium [15,16,17].

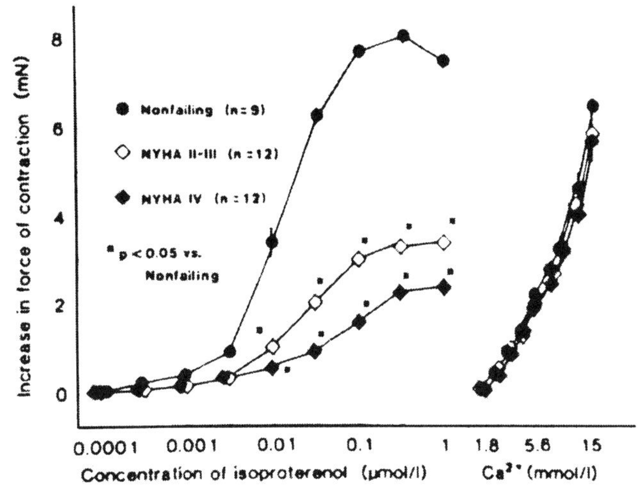

*Figure 11: Dose-response curves of left ventricular myocardium to isoproterenol **(left)** and calcium **(right)**. Nonfailing human myocardium is most sensitive to isoproterenol, whereas end-stage failing myocardium shows only little response. No difference was found regarding the response to calcium. According to [17].*

In addition, in myocardium from end-stage failing human hearts, a negative force-frequency relation has been described [5,18,19,20,21] (see Figure 12).

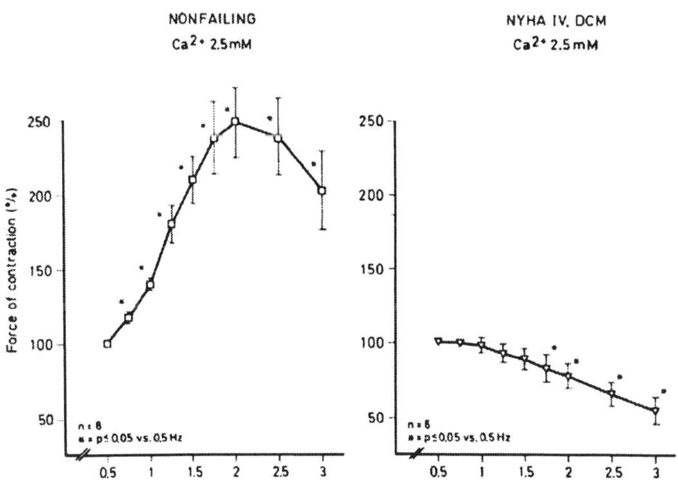

Figure 12: Force-Frequency relation is positive in nonfailing left ventricular myocardium, but negative in end-stage failing human myocardium.

In contrast to atrial human myocardium and other mammalian species, angiotensin II has no positive inotropic effect in human left ventricular myocardium [10]. However, endothelin has a mild positive inotropic effect on left ventricular human myocardium, an effect which is partially reduced in failing myocardium and possibly brought about by sensitization of the contractile proteins due to alkalization [22,23] (see also chapter VII).

3.2. Afterloaded Contractions

3.2.1. Animal Studies: Acute Interventions

A typical experiment in which the muscle is allowed to shorten against a series of different afterloads is shown in Figure 13.

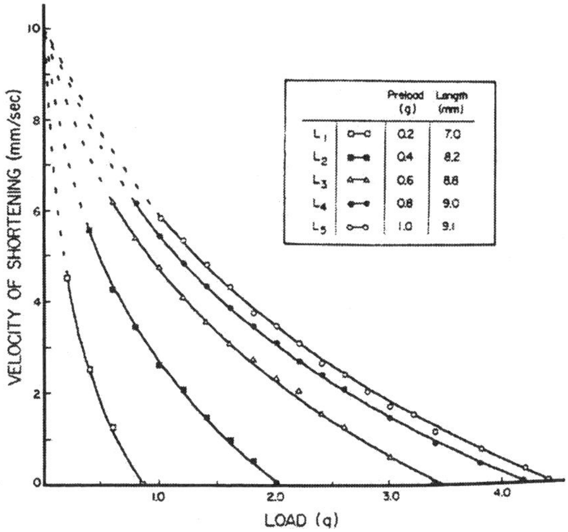

Figure 13: Force-velocity relations obtained from isolated right cat papillary muscle. Stimulation rate was constant 30/min, experimental temperature was 23.5°C. A family of curves was obtained which were extrapolated to a common intersection on the ordinate, i.e., V_{max}, maximum velocity of shortening. According to [7].

From the data presented in Figure 2, the following physical parameters can be derived: Velocity, extent of shortening and power (force multiplied by velocity) (see Figure 2). Changing preload, a family of force-velocity curves can be obtained (Figure 13). Extrapolation to zero load yields maximum shortening velocity V_{max}. According to Hill, the force-frequency relation can be described by a hyperbolic function using the following equation :

$$(P+a)\ V = b\ (P_0-P).$$

V_{max} could not only be analyzed by eye-ball extrapolation, but also by geometrical or mathematical means. Sonnenblick [6] analyzed the influence of acute interventions on force-velocity relations in the following way (Figure 14):

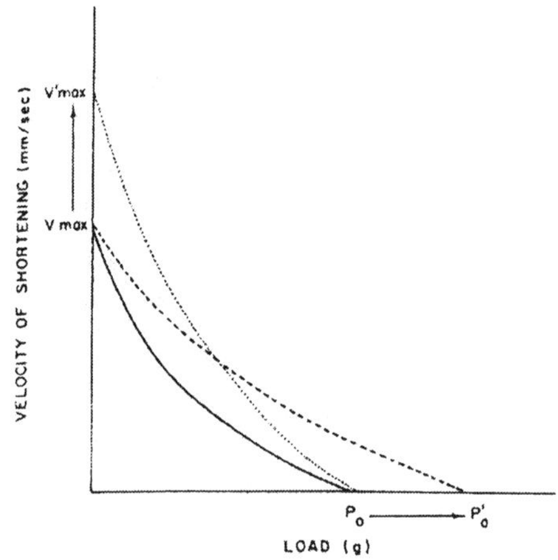

EFFECTS OF INTERVENTIONS ON THE FORCE VELOCITY RELATIONS OF THE CAT PAPILLARY MUSCLE

	V max	Po
INCREASING LENGTH	—	↑↑
INCREASING RATE	↑	↑ or —
NOREPINEPHRINE	↑↑	↑

Figure 14: Different effects of length, stimulation rate and norepinephrine on V_{max} and maximum developed force. According to [6].

3.2.2. Animal Studies: Chronic Changes

Cardiac hypertrophy and failure have been shown to be associated with a decrease in maximum shortening velocity (V_{max}) in a number of experimental models and species:

authors		species	model	V_{max}
Alpert et al.	[24]	rabbit	pulmonary banding	↓
Alpert et al.	[25]	rat	age	↓
Spann et al.	[11]	cat	pulmonary banding	↓
Jacob et al.	[26]	rat	Golblatt	↓
	[27]	rat	SHR	↓
	[28]	rat	aortic banding	↓
Ebrecht et al.	[29]	rat	hypothyroid	↓
Buccino et al.	[30]	cat	hypothyroid	↓

3.2.3. Human Studies: Acute Interventions

To our knowledge, force-velocity relations have not been published for human myocardial tissue. To study crossbridge kinetics in human cardiac tissues, more advanced technologies have been used like the frequency response method (see Chapter VI).

We have studied afterloaded contractions in human cardiac muscle tissue regarding the question whether positive inotropic compounds may have different influence on force development versus the extent of shortening [31]. Interestingly, a highly significant linear correlation with a slope close to unity was found between the fractional effect on shortening versus the fractional effect on force development, despite the use of four very different pharmacological modes of action: High calcium, isoproterenol, ouabain, and the calcium sensitizer EMD 570331 (see Figure 15) [31].

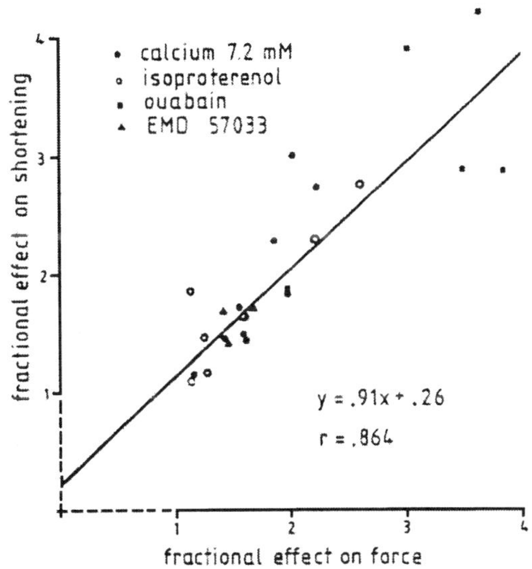

Figure 15: Effect of four different positive inotropic interventions on extent of shortening (ordinate) and on increase in force development (abscissa). A significant linear relationship was found with a slope close to unity. EMD 57033 is a pure calcium sensitizer. According to [31].

3.2.4. Human Studies: Chronic Changes

Again, no force-velocity relations of failing and non-failing human myocardium are available. However, there cannot be any doubt that maximum shortening velocity would have been found to be reduced, because more advanced technologies have demonstrated slowed crossbridge dynamics (see Chapter VI, frequency response method).

We have studied afterloaded contractions in human failing versus non-failing muscle preparations, because muscle length and stimulation frequency may have different effects on the extent of shortening versus the effect on force development, and thereby on work performance. We found that the Frank-Starling mechanism is preserved in human failing myocardium regarding both force development and work performed [31]. Furthermore, the negative force-frequency relationship in failing human myocardium results in a negative work-frequency relation: However, the relative effects of frequency modulation on work performance are much greater (at least by a factor of 2) than on force development (Figure 16) [31].

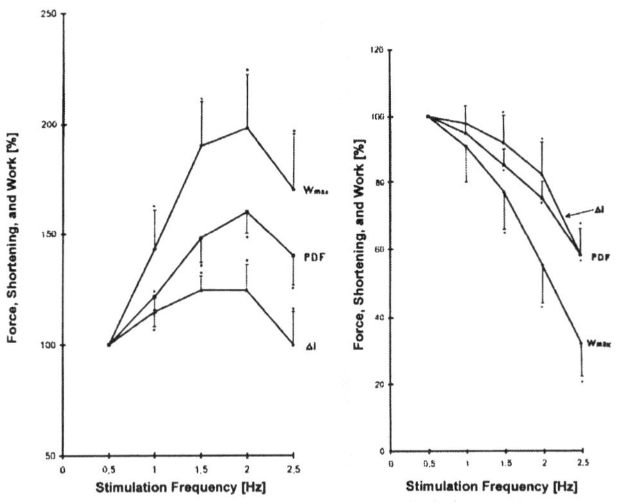

*Figure 16: Influence of stimulation frequency on peak developed force (PDF), extent of shortening (Δl), and maximum work (W_{max}) in nonfailing **(left)** and failing **(right)** human ventricular muscle preparations. (1) Effects are positive in nonfailing but negative in failing myocardium. (2) Effects are most pronounced regarding maximum work (W_{max}). According to [31].*

3.4. Discussion

In order to describe completely the mechanical properties of a muscle (skeletal or cardiac), experiments and measurements must be conducted that allow constructions of length-tension relations as well as force-velocity relations. As shown in the Results section, acute interventions and chronic molecular alterations may differently influence these relations. In this context, rat Goldblatt model may be of special interest, because maximum shortening velocity was decreased (due to heavy chain myosin composition), whereas peak systolic force was increased (due to a greater density of muscle proteins). Despite these physiological basic facts, the initial "V_{max}"-concept was greatly overestimated. The idea was to determine (extrapolate) the maximum shortening velocity "V_{max}" in vitro and in vivo. Since, in 1962, Sonnenbick had shown that "V_{max}" was preload-independent (Figure 14) [6], V_{max} was thought to be an ideal parameter to measure "contractility". It took several years to find out that this "one and only" parameter is not suited as a general index – especially in the clinical situation. Nevertheless, for many years V_{max} has helped to analyze experimentally molecular alterations of the myocardium which take place during cardiac hypertrophy and failure: Reduced contraction velocity has been attributed to shifts of the α- and β-myosin heavy chain composition (even in man) [32], the troponin-T isoforms [33], and also the phosphorylation site of myosin light chains [34].

Furthermore, measurements of "V_{max}" by force-velocity relations and respective extrapolation are hampered by the fact that the active state of the muscle, i.e., the activation of the contractile proteins by calcium, influences the experimental measurements. Therefore, it is likely that changes in calcium and heart rate (see Figure 14) do not influence intrinsic shortening velocity like for example norepinephrine, but rather alter excitation-contraction coupling, and thereby the active state.

Therefore, to detect alterations of basic mechanisms, more sophisticated measurements were developed (myothermal method, skinned fiber, frequency response method, see Chapters IV, V, VI).

On the other hand, isolated muscle preparations have brought many new insights into pathophysiological and molecular alterations of the human diseased heart simply by isometric measurements and length-tension diagrams, most importantly, the β-adrenoceptor downregulation (see Figure 9) [15,16,17] and the reversed force-frequency relation (see Figure 10) [18,19,20,21].

One other aspect, which has not yet been mentioned in this chapter, is diastolic compliance. When constructing length-tension diagrams, the passive elastic properties are determined as well. However, the whole chapter VIII is dedicated to diastolic compliance.

REFERENCES

1) Mulieri LA, Ittleman F, Blanchard EM, Alpert NR: Protection of human left ventricular myocardium from cutting injury with 2,3-butanedione monoxime. Circ Res, 1989. 65:1441-1444

2) Holubarsch Ch, Blanchard EM, Alpert NR, Mulieri LA, Just H: Myothermal economy of rat myocardium, chronic adaptation versus acute inotropism. 1986, Darmstadt: Dr. Steinkopff Verlag. 95-101

3) Hasenfuss G, Blanchard EM, Holubarsch C, Leavitt BJ, Ittleman F, Alpert NR: Energetics of isometric force development in control and volume overload human myocardium: comparison with animal species. Circ Res, 1991. 68:836-846

4) Paradise NF, Surmitis JM: Criteria for adequate oxygenation of isometric kitten papillary muscle. Am J Physiol, 1981. 241:H348-H353

5) Mulieri LA, Leavitt B, Allen PD, Alpert NR: Altered myocardial force-frequency relation in human heart failure. Circulation, 1992. 85:1743-1750

6) Sonnenblick E: Implications of muscle mechanics in the heart. Fed Proc, 1962. 21:975-990

7. Sonnenblick E: Force-velocity relations in mammalian heart muscle. Am J Physiol, 1962. 202:931-939

8) Bowditch H: Über die Eigentümlichkeiten der Reizbarkeit welche Muskelfasern des Herzens zeigen. Ber Sachs Ges Akkad, 1871. 23: 652-689

9) Koch-Weser J: Myocardial action of angiotensin. Circ Res, 1964. 14:337-343

10. Holubarsch Ch, Schmidt-Schweda S, Knorr H, Pieske B, Ruf T, Fasol R, Just H: Angiotensin I and II exert inotropic effects in atrial but not in ventricular human myocardium. Circulation, 1993. 88: 1228-1237

11) Spann JF, Eckberg KL, Sonnenblick EH, Ross J, Braunwald E: Contractile performance of the hypertrophied and chronically failing cat ventricle. Am J Physiol, 1972. 223: 1150-1157

12) Holubarsch Ch, Jacob R, Medugorac I, Thiedemann K-U: Passive elastic properties of myocardium in different models and stages of hypertrophy: Astudy comparing mechanical, chemical, and morphometric parameters., in Myocardial Hypertrophy and Failure., A. NR, Editor. 1983, Raven Press: New York:323-335

13) Bing OH, Brooks WW, Conrad CH, Sen S, Perreault CL, Morgan JP: Intracellular calcium transients in myocardium from spontaneously hypertensive rats during the transition to heart failure. Circ Res 1991 68(5):1390-400

14) Holubarsch Ch, Golstein DJ, Ashton RC, Nickl W, Pieske B, Pioch K, Lüdemann J, Wiesner S, Hasenfuss G, Posival H, Just H, Burkhoff D: Existence of the Frank-Starling mechanism in the failing human heart. Circulation, 1996. 94: 683-689

15) Bristow MR, Ginsburg R, Minobe WA, Cubicciotti RS, Sageman WS, Lurie K, Billingham MR, Harrison DL, Stinson EB: Decreased catecholamine sensitivity and beta-adrenergicreceptor density in failing human hearts. New England J Med 1982;307:205-211

16) Brodde O: ß1- and ß2-adrenoceptors in the human heart: properties, function and alterations in chronic heart failure. Pharmacol Rev, 1991. 43: 202-242

17) Böhm M, Pieske B, et al.: Contribution of cAMP-phosphorylation inhibition and sensitization of the contractile proteins for calcium to the inotropic effect of pimobendan in th failing human myocardium. Circ Res, 1991. 68:689-701

18) Feldman MD, Phillips P, Schoen F, Morgan JP: Reversal of the force-frequency relationship in working myocardium from patients with endstage heart filure. J Appl Cardiol, 1988. 3: 273-283

19) Pieske B, Holubarsch C, Schwinger R, Böhm M, Just H: Alteration of the force-frequency relationship in the failing human heart depends on underlying disease. Basic Res Cardiol, 1992. 87(Suppl3): 213-221

20) Hasenfuss G, Studer R, Meyer M, Pieske B, Holtz J, Holubarsch Ch, Posival H, Just H, Drexler H: Relation between myocardial function and expression of sarcoplasmic reticulum Ca2+-ATPase in failing and nonfailing human myocardium. Circ Res, 1994. 75: 434-442

21) Holubarsch Ch, Pieske B, Ruf T, Hasenfuss G, Fraedrich G, Posival H, Just H: Positive and negative inotropic effect of DL-Sotalol and D-Sotalol in failing and nonfailing human myocardium under physiological experimental conditions. Circulation, 1995. 92: 2904-2910

22) Holubarsch Ch, Kretschmann B, Schmidt-Schweda S, Meyer M, Schlotthauer K, Ruf T, Hasenfuss G, Just H: The functional role of angiotensin and endothelin in failing and nonfailing human myocardium., in The failing Heart, B.R. Dhalla NS, Takeda N, Nagano M, Editor. 1995, Lippincott-Raven Publishers: Philadelphia

23) Pieske B, Bren V, Löffler B, Schlotthauer K, Maier L, Schmidt-Schweda S, Just H, Hasenfuss G: Functional effects of endothelin and regulation of endothelin receptors in isolated human non-failing and failing myocardium. Circulation, 1999. 99: 1802-1809

24) Alpert NR, Holpern W: Mechanical and biochemical correlates of cardiac hypertrophy. Circ Res, 1974. 34&35(Suppl2): 71-82

25) Alpert NR, Taylor N, The effect of age on contractile protein, ATPase activity and the velocity of shortening., in Factors influencing myocardial contractility., K.F. Tanz RD, Roberts J, Editor. 1967, Acedemic Press: New York. 127-133

26) Jacob R, Kämmereit A, Medugorac I, Wendt-Gallitelli MF: Myocardial function in different models of cardiac hypertrophy. An attempt at correlating mechanical, biochemical and morphological parameters. Basic Res Cardiol, 1977. 72: 160-166

27) Jacob R, Erbrecht G, Holubarsch Ch, Medugorac J: Elastic and contractile properties of the myocardium in experimental cardiac hypertrophy of the rat. Methodological and pathophysiological considerations. Basic Res Cardiol 1980; 75: 253-261

28) Jacob R, Holubarsch C, Rupp H, Kissling G: Mechanics and energetics in cardiac hypertrophy as related to the isoenzyme pattern of myosin., in Perspectives in Cardiovascular Research: Myocardial Hypertrophy and Failure., A. NR, Editor. 1983, Raven Press: New York. 553-570

29) Ebrecht G, Jacob R: Alterations of mechanical parameters in chemically skinned preparations of rat myocardium as a functional of isoenzyme pattern of myosin. Basic Res Cardiol, 1982. 77: 220-234

30) Buccino RA, Pool PE: Sonnenblick EH, Braunwald E: Influence of the thyroid state on the intrinsic contractile properties and energy stores of the myocardium. J Clin Invest, 1967. 46: 1669-1682

31) Holubarsch Ch, Wiessner S, Ruf Th, Schulte-Baukloh H, Schmidt-Schweda S, Pieske B, Posival H, Just H: Shortening versus isometric contractions in isolated human hailing and non-failing left ventricular myocardium. Dependency of external work and force on muscle length, heart rate and inotropic stimulation. Cardiovasc Res, 1998. 37: 46-57

32) Lowes Bd, Abraham WT, et al: Changes in gene expression in the intact human heart. Downregulation of α-myosin heavy chain in hypertrophied, failing ventricular myocardium. J Clin Invest, 1997. 100: 2315-2324

33) Anderson PAW, Oakelay AF, Pagani ED, Allen PD: Troponin T isoform expression in humans. A comparison among normal and failing adult heart, fetal heart, and adult and fetal skeletal muscle. Circ Res, 1991. 69: 1226-1233

34) Morano I: Effects of different expression and posttranslational modifications of myosin light chains on contractility of skinned human cardiac fibers. Basic Res Cardiol, 1992. 87(Suppl1): 129-141

4. THE MYOTHERMAL APPROACH

4.1. Introduction

An introduction to the myothermal approach is given in Chapter II: The Myothermal Method: Historical and Personal Aspects.

4.2. Methods

The measurements of rapid heat output of small-dimensioned cardiac muscle preparations (about 5 mm long and 0.5 mm in thickness) are based on the principle of thermocouples and thermopiles. When two wires existing of two different metals are soldered at both their ends to a unit ring, a thermocouple results (Figure 1).

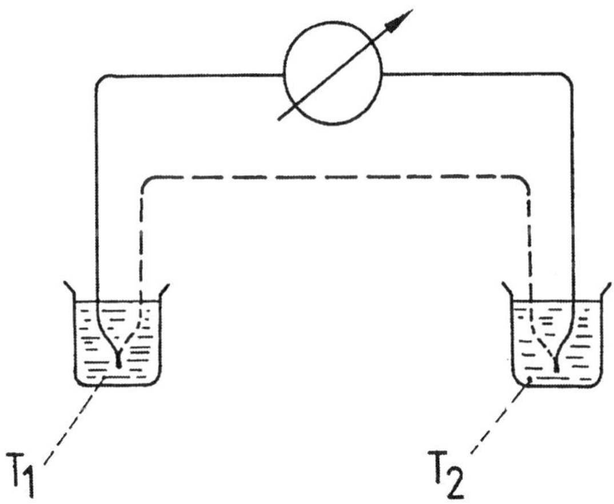

Figure 1: The principle of myothermal method: A thermocouple composed of two different metals (— and ----). See text.

If both connecting ends are exposed to different temperatures, a thermovoltage is generated and can be measured according to the following equation:

$$\eta = \frac{\Delta U_{therm}}{\Delta T} = a + 2b\,(T1 - T2)$$

when η is the electromotive force, ΔU_{therm} is the voltage change induced by the temperature difference ΔT, a and b are constants, and T1 and T2 are the respective absolute temperatures [1]. For some metal combinations, b is roughly zero – at least in small temperature intervals – so that η equals the constant a or, in other words, the thermovoltage ΔU_{therm} is directly proportional to the temperature difference ΔT. A number of those thermocouples adjusted in series is called a thermopile (Figure 2).

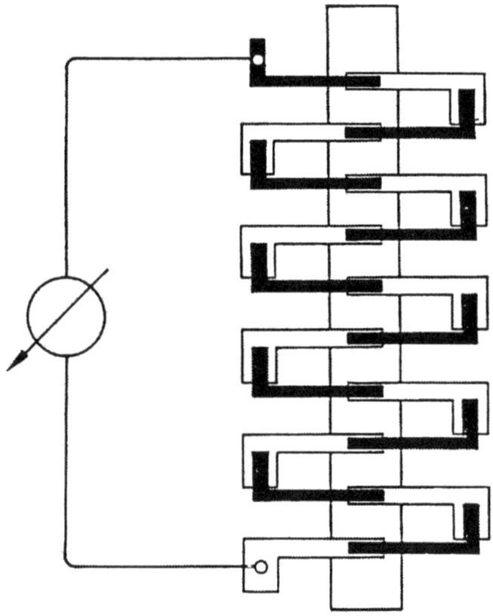

Figure 2: The principle of a thermopile: A number of thermocouples is located in series. If the central junctions of the two different metals (black and white) is heated and the temperature of the peripheral junctions maintained at constant temperature, a voltage output can be measured which is proportional to the number of central junctions and the heat liberated by a longitudinal muscle preparation which is in contact with the central junctions (see text).

In such a system, thermovoltages ΔU_{therm} of the single thermocouples are added, if the central so-called active junctions are at higher temperature T2 and the peripheral so-called reference junctions are at lower temperature T1. One can easily depict from Figure 2 that a longitudinal cylindrically shaped muscle preparation positioned on the active junctions will increase the temperature of these junctions by heat liberation, whereas the peripheral reference junctions are kept at constant temperature. The measured voltage change is therefore a function of (1) the electromotive force of a single junction, (2) the temperature difference ΔT created by the heat liberation of the muscle, and (3) the number of the active junctions.

In order to measure by means of this myothermal principle temperature changes induced by a cardiac muscle preparation, the thermopile has to be isolated electrically without blocking or retarding the thermal conductance between muscle and metals. For this purpose, extremely breakable thinnest mica sheets were used [2,3,4]. In order to use this principle of temperature measurements also in small-dimensioned papillary muscles or trabeculae of the myocardium, construction of thermopiles with lowest electrical resistance and optimally high electromotive force of the whole system are needed. Mulieri et al. [5] resolved this problem by using antimony and bismuth, two metals that could not be used before because of their brittleness, but exhibit the highest electromotive force possible [1,2]. Using high vacuum evaporation methods, the first metal was deposited by means of a copper template on a 5-8 μm thick sheet. Thereafter, the template was turned by 180° and the other metal was deposited by vacuum evaporation in a mirror-like manner. A second mica sheet was then used to cover the metal layers in a sandwich-like manner, and the thermopile was sealed by an isolation glue.

The thermopiles we used in Burlington/Vermont/USA had 20 active junctions allowing to use either all of them or only 14 for shorter muscle preparations. The thickness of a thermopile was about 20 μm, and temperature sensitivity was in the magnitude of 1 to 1.5 mV/°C as measured according to the method of Hill and Woledge [6]. Thermal capacity was 0.3 mcal/°C, and heat loss coefficient was 0.535 mcal/°C sec. These parameters were determined by a modified method of Kretschmer and Wilkie [7]. Instead of heating silver strips positioned on the thermopile with Peltier effect, in Burlington we heated the silver strips by means of infrared diodes (Figure 3).

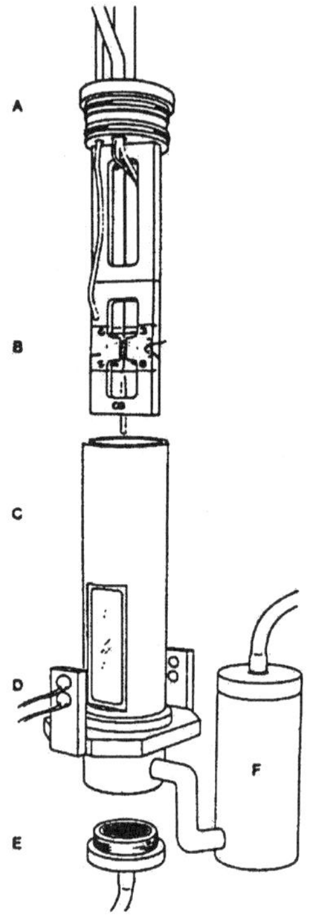

Figure 3: The complete thermopile apparatus: ***A.*** *Head of thermopile frame with two rubber O-ring seal.* ***B.*** *Thermopile metal frame.* ***C.*** *Stainless steel muscle chamber with glass windows.* ***D.*** *Infrared diodes on both sides of the window.* ***E.*** *Bottom of muscle chamber with fritted steel disk for gassing.* ***F.*** *The solution reservoir.* According to [5].

Cardiac muscle preparations were prepared as described in Chapter III. However, instead of using the clipping methods (metal forceps) or steel hooks for connections between muscle and instruments, only non-metal connecting systems were allowed in myothermal experiments. Therefore, the ends of muscle preparations were carefully fixed to silk ligatures which contained 20 μm thin platinum wires by means of which an end-to-end electrical stimulation of the muscle preparation was provided (Figure 4B).

One ligature was hooked to a fixed lower glass hook (isometric contraction), the other to a long upper glass stylus (30 cm), which was attached to a capacitance-type-force-transducer [8]. According to Figure 4, the cylindrical muscle preparation is thereby attached to the active junctions of the thermopile. An additional tether-like silk ligature was stretched on the lower ligature in order to guarantee a good contact between the muscle and thermopile (Figure 4).

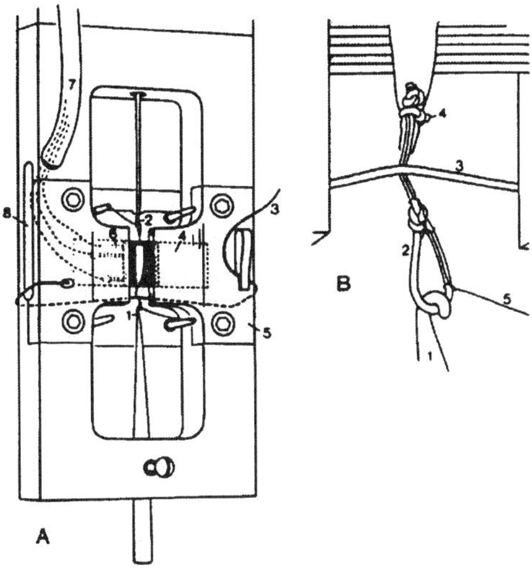

*Figure 4: **A:** The thermopile in details: 1) Lower glas stylus. 2) Upper glas stylus connected to a force transducer. 3) Tether to fix the muscle preparation in good contact with the thermopile. 4) and 6) Reference junctions of the thermopile. 5) Removeable part of the metal frame (necessary for thermopile exchange). 7) Wire connections from thermopile to amplifier. 8) Access ports.*
***B:** The lower end of the muscle: 1) Lower glas stylus. 2) Silk loop. 3) Tether. 4) Silk ligature. 5) Platinum wire for stimulation.*

The solutions used are described in Chapter III. The preparations mounted on the thermopile were submerged into Krebs-Ringer solution which was bubbled by a gas mixture of 95 % O_2 and 5 % CO_2. Before heat measurements could be performed, the solution had to be drained into a reservoir chamber (F in Figure 3). During that experimental period, the surrounding of the muscle preparation was constantly passed by a moisturized mixture of 95 % O_2 and 5 % CO_2. Under those conditions, the temperature of the thermopile directly reflects the heat output of the muscle liberated at a faster and a slower rate as shown in Figure 5.

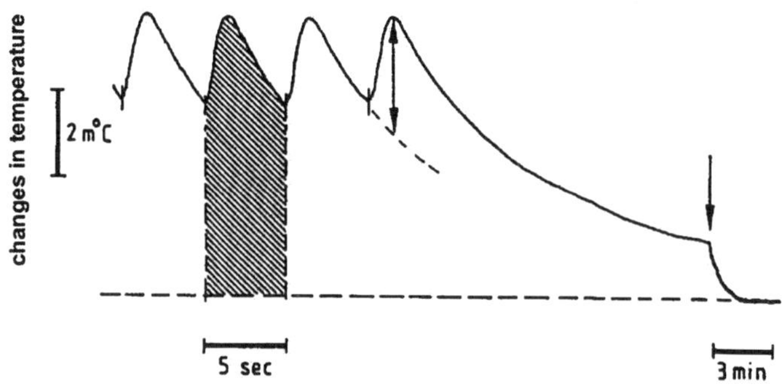

Figure 5: Original temperature record: The oscillating heat signal results from continuous stimulation of a muscle preparation at 0.2 Hz. Initial heat is calculated from the temperature difference between peak temperature and extrapolation of the experimental cool-off curve of the preceeding twitch (arrow). Total activity-related heat is the area between the oscillating temperature signal and the baseline for one twitch interval (5 sec; cross-hatched area).

The heat that is liberated fast is called initial heat and is represented by the distance between peak temperature and the extrapolated cool-off of the proceeding twitch (arrow in Figure 5). Total activity-related heat is called all the heat – whether liberated fast or slow – during a twitch interval as given by the temperature-time area between the temperature signal and baseline during one twitch (5 sec in the experiment shown in Figure 5). Total activity-related heat is the sum of initial heat which is associated with force generation and recovery heat which is related to the resynthesis of ATP from glucose and oxygen (Figures 6 and 8).

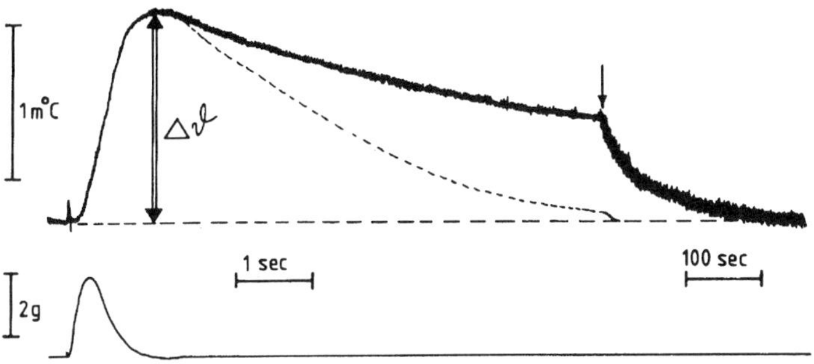

Figure 6: A single twitch experiment for demonstration of analysis of initial heat, recovery heat, and total activity-related heat. The fast increase in the temperature signal ($\Delta\vartheta$, see arrow) is due to initial heat liberation, i.e., ATP splitting during contraction. Therefore, initial heat can be derived from initial temperature change $\Delta\vartheta$, the cool-off constant τ, and the heat loss coefficient. The slow heat release starts at the peak of the temperature signal and is reflected by the area between the two cool-off lines: --- hypothetical cool-off curve of initial heat. ~~~ measured cool-off curve of total activity-related heat. Total activity-related heat can be derived from the whole area underneath the measured heat signal (from begin to the end of heat release) and the heat loss coefficient. Recovery heat (from ATP resynthesis) is simply the difference between total activity-related heat and initial heat (see also Figure 8).

Initial heat can be further divided into tension-dependent heat (TDH) which is the heat due to ATP splitting of the actomyosin system (cross-bridge cycling) and tension-independent heat (TIH) which is the heat due to ATP splitting used for Ca^{2+} pumping (Figures 7 and 8).

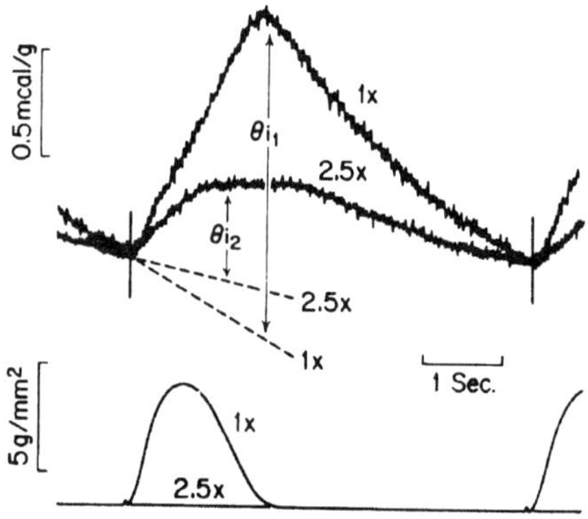

Figure 7: Experimental separation between tension-dependent heat (TDH) and tension-independent heat (TIH). In this Figure, the mannitol method is demonstrated: Addition of mannitol (2.5x) to the solution eliminates active tension development ***(lower trace)*** *thereby eliminates TDH. Initial heat* ***(upper trace)*** *can be calculated from the temperature signal of the untreated muscle (1x), and the TIH from the temperature signal of the mannitol treated muscle (2.5x; upper trace). TDH is simply the subtraction of TIH from initial heat. According to [29].*

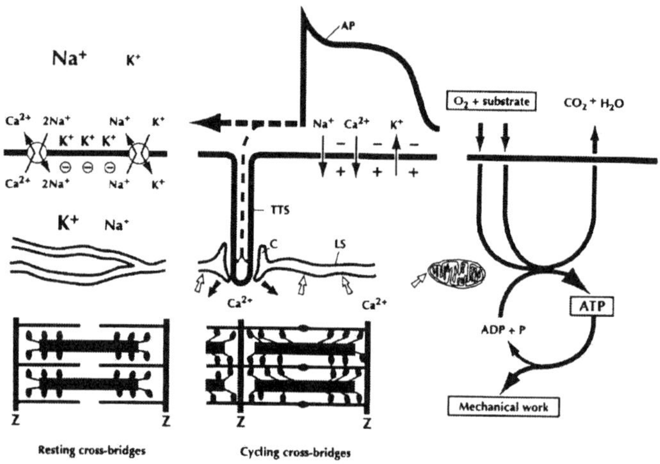

Figure 8: Demonstration of the different heat components as illustrated in a cardiac muscle cell. ***Left:*** *Resting heat rate (see Figure 9) is composed of energetic process involved in some crossbridge cycling at rest, protein synthesis, and ion pumping enzymes being active at rest.* ***Middle:*** *Initial heat is composed of energy consumption process in calcium turnover (see Figure 7) and of energy turnover of the actomyosin system (tension-dependent heat).* ***Right:*** *Demonstration of recovery heat process: Regeneration of ATP from oxygen and glucose (see Figure 6).*

If the muscle is not stimulated, the resting muscle releases the resting heat which can be measured by submerging the muscle into temperature-equilibrated solution (Figure 9).

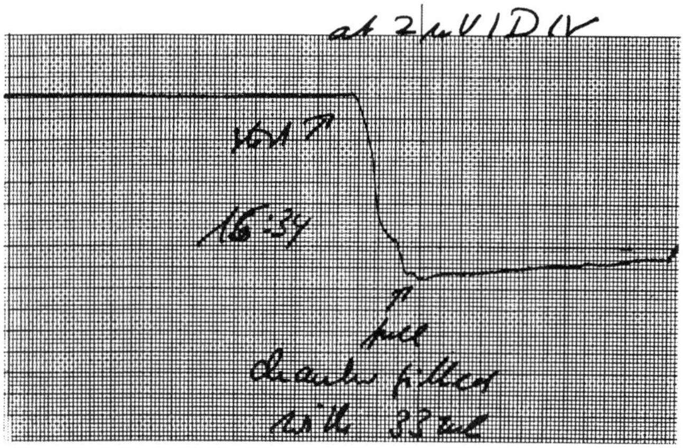

Figure 9: Original record for measuring resting heart rate: The muscle preparation is abruptly (start-full) submerged into temperature-equilibrated solution. The drop in temperature represents resting heat rate.

The resting heat may come from three different sources: (1) Cycling cross-bridges at diastole, (2) protein synthesis, (3) ion pumping enzymes being active also at rest to maintain the ion milieu. A summary of all the different heat components is shown in Figure 8.

4.3. Results

Results obtained with the myothermal method are separated into four sections: A. Acute changes in energetics of animal myocardium. B. Chronic changes in energetics of animal myocardium. C. Acute changes of energetics of human myocardium. D. Chronic changes in energetics of human myocardium.

4.3.1. Acute Changes of Energetics in Animal Myocardium

The strength of the heart beat is under the permanent physiological control of at least four important mechanisms. (1) Preload and therefore muscle fiber length determines the force of contraction (Frank-Starling) [9,10]. (2) Heart frequency has influence on force of contraction (Treppe) [11]. (3) The sympathetic tone via the release of noradrenaline (or adrenaline) controls not only peripheral resistance but also contractility via stimulation of myocardial β_1- and β_2-adrenoceptors. (4) Angiotensin and endothelin may exert positive inotropic effects [13]. Furthermore, positive inotropic compounds are used acutely and chronically to support the failing heart. Understanding the mode of action of these interventions and their influence on myocardial energetics is essential for treatment of patients and development of new therapeutic strategies. The most economic way of an acute increase in force generation is an increase in fiber length (sarcomere length), a mechanism which was first described by Frank and Starling (see Chapter I). Because increase in force generation is induced by a length-dependent sensitization of the contractile proteins to calcium, no extra energy is needed for the handling of extra calcium neither for the transport from the cytosol to the saroplasmic reticulum nor from the cytosol to the extracellular space (Chapter I).

Measurements of tension-dependent heat and tension-independent heat (= activation heat) depend on our ability to partition the initial heat into its components. Two different methods have been used for evaluation of activation heat: The shortening method [4,14] and BDM method [15]. The shortening method has been criticized for two reasons: (1) At a short length, extra heat may be released by cycling cross-bridges without virtual force development. (2) At short muscle length, the membrane releases less calcium than at l_{max}, i.e., activation heat is not constant but rather length-dependent. On the other hand, the BDM-method may also be critical, because at higher doses of BDM not only cross-bridge interaction and thereby tension-dependent heat may be blocked but also the calcium release and thereby activation heat may be influenced [16]. Therefore, we have performed a study in which we compared activation heat measured with both methods in a variety of muscles and conditions (Figure 10) [17]. A good linear correlation was found with a slope of 0.6l indicating that the shortening method may somewhat overestimate activation heat [17].

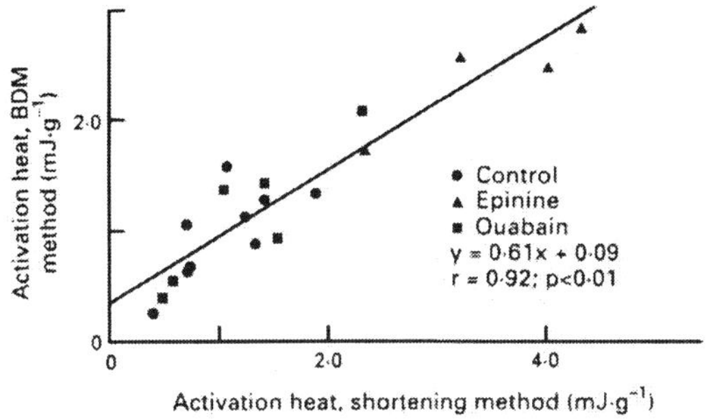

Figure 10: Activation heat, i.e., tension-independent heat, as analyzed by either the shortening method (abszissa) or the BDM method (ordinate, see text). Although there is a significant correlation, the shortening method may overestimate or the BDM method may underestimate activation heat. According to [17].

We investigated two substances that are known to stimulate β_1- and β_2-adrenoceptors: Isoproterenol and Epinine. For comparison, we also studied the influence of high calcium and ouabain, as well as the phosphodiesterase inhibitor E-1020. Pimobendan, one of the first calcium-sensitizers was also included in this study [17,18,19]. Original records are depicted in Figure 11 for a typical experiment.

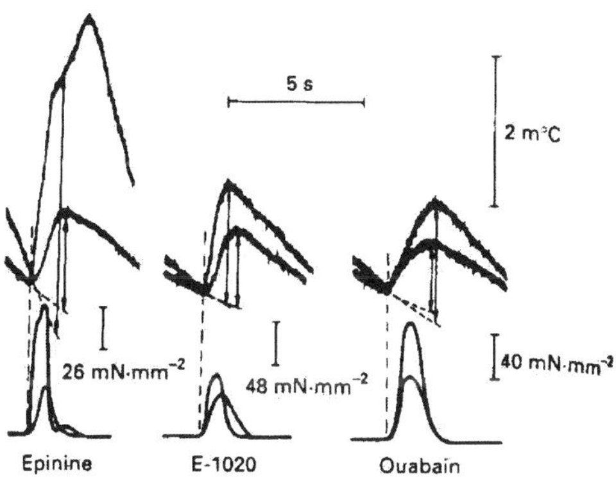

*Figure 11: Original records for force development **(lower trace)** and heat production **(upper trace)** in guinea pig papillary muscle treated with epinin (β_1-adrenoceptor agonist, left), E-1020 (phosphodiesterase inhibitor, middle), and ouabain (digitalis, right). The most economical positive inotropic intervention is ouabain: Large increase in force production (force-time integral), but small increase in heat output. According to [17].*

Quantitative and statistical analysis of activation heat (tension-independent heat) are given in Figure 12 and the relation between tension-time integral and tension-dependent heat are given in Figure 13.

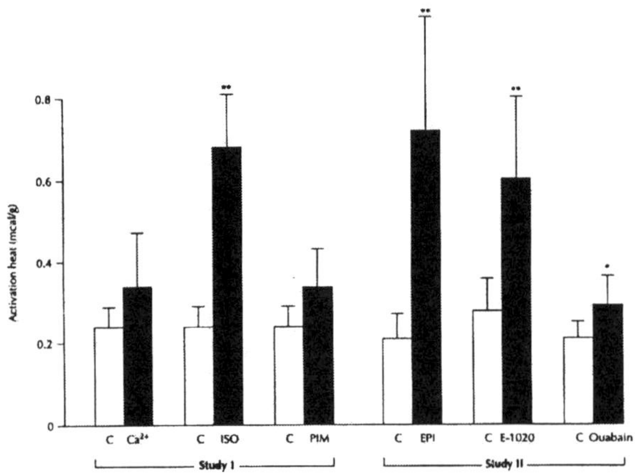

Figure 12: Activation heat, i.e., tension-independent heat, in two studies with positive inotropic interventions. ***Study I:*** *High calcium, Ca^{2+}; Isoproterenol, ISO; Pimobendan, PIM.* ***Study II:*** *Epinine, EPI; Phosphodiesterase-inhibition, E-1020; Digitalis, Ouabain. According to [19].*

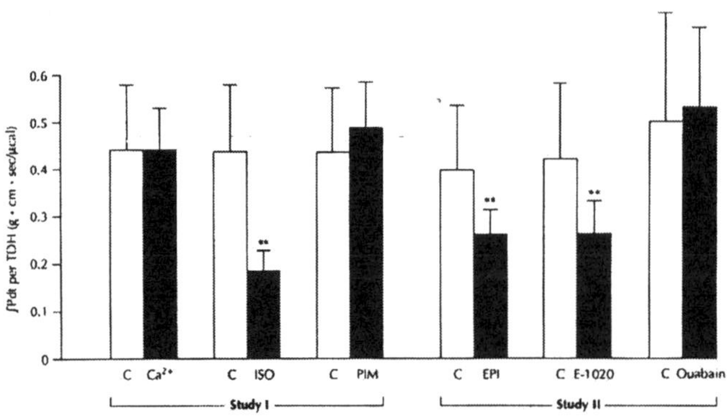

Figure 13: Economy of myocardial contraction on the level of the contractile proteins as analyzed from tension-time integral (∫Pdt) and tension-dependent heat (TDH) in two studies with positive inotropic interventions. ***Study I:*** *High calcium, Ca^{2+}: No change; Isoproterenol, ISO: Decrease; Pimobendane, PIM: No change.* ***Study II:*** *Epinine, EPI: Decrease; Phosphodiesterase inhibitor, E-1020: Decrease; Digitalis, Ouabain: No change. According to [19].*

From the data in Figure 13, the force-time integral of a single cross-bridge can be calculated under the following assumptions:

(1) ∫ PdtM / TDH ½ sarcomere = ∫ PdtCB / ΔH molecule ATP
(2) ∫ PdtCB = ∫ PdtM / TDH ½ sarcomere * ΔH molecule ATP

when ∫ PdtM is the tension-time integral of the muscle, ∫ PdtCB is the tension-time integral of a single cross-bridge, TDH ½ sarcomere is the tension-dependent heat of the muscle for half a sarcomere, and ΔH molecule ATP equals the enthalpy of one molecule of ATP. One has to be aware that two assumptions are being made when creating these equations: One molecule of ATP is split per cross-bridge cycle, and the tension-time integral of the muscle is the sum of the force-time integrals of all cross-bridges. The calculated cross-bridge force-time integral under the different pharmacological conditions is given in Figure 14.

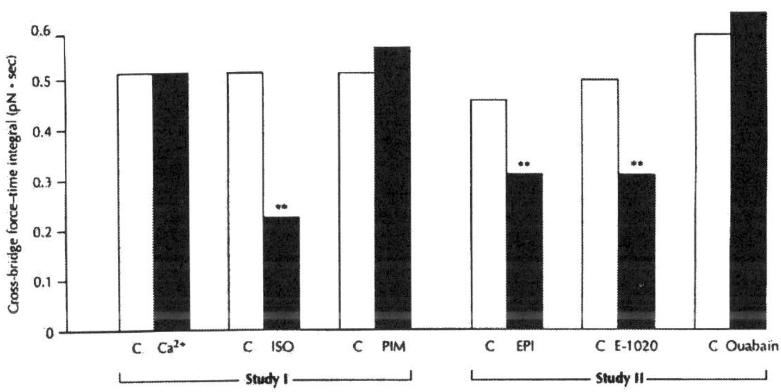

*Figure 14: Calculated crossbridge force-time integral of a single crossbridge, in two studies with positive inotropic interventions. **Study I:** High calcium, Ca^{2+}: No change; Isoproterenol, ISO: Decrease; Pimobendan, PIM: No change. **Study II:** Epinine, EPI: Decrease; Phosphodiesterase inhibition, E-1020: Decrease; Digitalis, Ouabain: No change. According to [19].*

Figures 12 and 13 indicate the different energetic consequences of the compounds used to stimulate the myocardium: Isoproterenol and epinine both compounds stimulate β_1-adrenoceptors triplicate activation heat as do phophodiesterase inhibitors. Therefore, these positive inotropic substances act mainly by a dramatic increase in the number of calcium ions cycled per beat. In contrast, high calcium, pimobendan and ouabain have only a small effect on activation heat.

In addition to the alteration in calcium cycling, the economy of force generation on the level of the contractile proteins is also altered by isoproterenol, epinine and phosphodiesterase inhibition. ∫ Pdt per TDH is half of control with these compounds (Figure 13) indicating a decrease in the cross-bridge force-time integral (Figure 14). In contrast, high calcium, pimbomendan and ouabain have no effect on mechanics and energetics of crossbridges.

Figure 15 shows a summary of the overall energetic consequences of positive inotropic compounds by plotting initial heat as a function of the tension-time integral: phosphodiesterase inhibition and β-adrenoceptor stimulation are the most uneconomical means to increase force of contraction. Ouabain, BAY8644, a calcium channel agonist, and high calcium indicate more economical stimulation of the myocardium. Pimobendan and especially EMD 53998, both calcium sensitizers, are the most economical means to increase force of contraction (Figure 15).

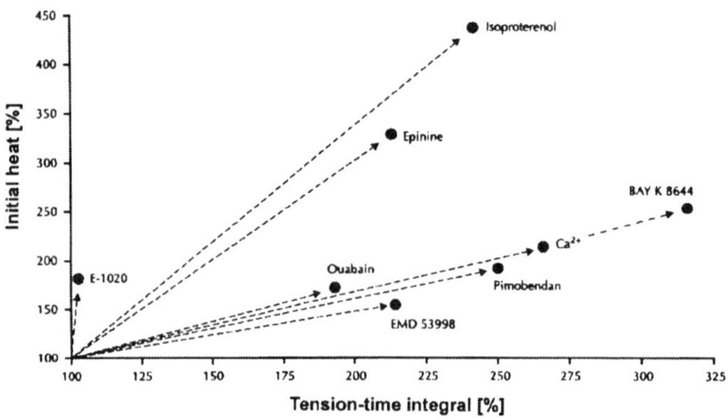

Figure 15: Relationship between the increase in initial heat and tension-time integral due to positive inotropic compounds. The steeper the slopes, the less economical the type of stimulation: Phosphodiesterase inhibitors (E-1020) and β_1-adrenoceptors agonists (isoproterenol and epinine) are uneconomical compared to the other positive inotropic compounds. The calcium-sensitizer EMD 53998 is the most economical way of positive inotropic stimulation.

4.3.2. Chronic Changes of Energetics in Animal Myocardium

It has been known for a long time that pressure overload leads to a reduction of myocardial contraction velocity (see Chapter III). Biochemical studies showed that reduced shortening velocity is associated with reduced myofibrillar ATPase activity [20,21,22]. The first authors who showed the basic molecular alterations for these important functional properties of the myocardium were Lompré et al. [23] for the pressure overloaded rat heart and Hoh and coworkers [24] for the hypothyrotic rat heart. Later on, it was shown that these shifts in the isoenzyme pattern of myosin (αα-homodimer, αβ-heterodimer, ββ-homodimer) also occur in diabetic rats [25]. It was of great interest to know in as far these fundamental changes in the molecular composition of the myosin heavy chains have impact on myocardial energetics. We therefore studied the correlation between myocardial energetics and the myosin isoenzyme pattern in Goldblatt rats (renal hypertension) [26,27] and hypothyrotic rats (rats treated with propylthiouracil (PTU) for three weeks) [28]. Experiments were performed using single twitches as well as tetanic contractions of different duration.

Changes of the isomyosin composition are shown in Figure 16 for PTU-treatment and for Goldblatt hypertension.

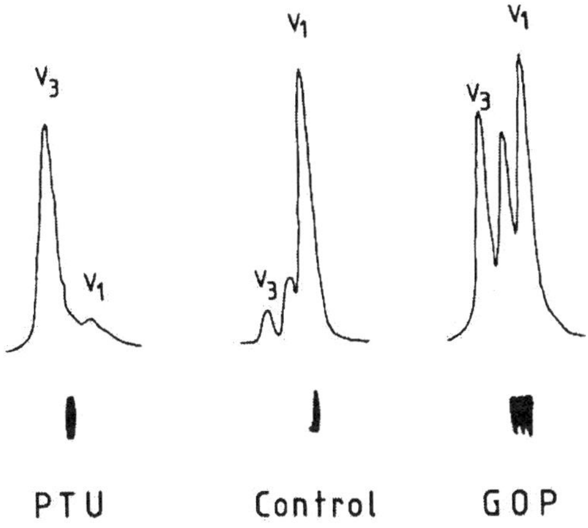

Figure 16: Myosin isoenzyme pattern of the young rat left ventricle: V_1 = αα homodimer, V_2 = αβ heterodimer, V_3 = ββ homodimer. In the control myocardium, V_1 myosin prevails, in Goldblatt hypertension (GOP) equal amounts of V_1, V_2, and V_3 exist, whereas in prophylthiouracil-treated (PTU), i.e., hypothyrotic rats, V_1 and V_2 almost completely disappeared.

Redistribution of V1 (αα-homodimers) towards V3 (ββ-homodimer) is almost complete in hypothyroidism but less pronounced in Goldblatt hypertension. In twitch contraction as well as in tetanic contraction, the shift in isoenzyme patterns improved economy of myocardial contraction: Figure 17 shows the ratio between heat and peak twitch tension or tension-time integral in diagram A and the slope of total-activity-related heat vs. tension-time integral in tetanic contractions.

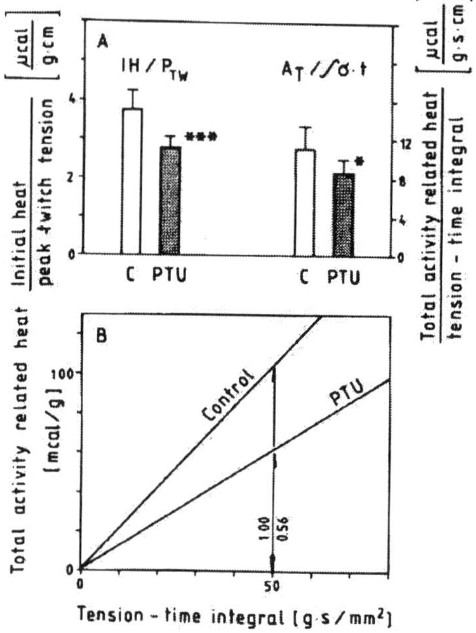

*Figure 17: Economy of myocardial contraction in prophylthiouracil treated rats in twitches **(A)** and tetanic contractions **(B)**. Economy of twitches is analyzed by either relating initial heat to peak twitch tension (IH/P_{TW}) on the left or relating total activity-related heat to tension-time integral ($A_T/\int\sigma t$) on the right. Both indices decrease in PTU as compared to C (control) indicating a better economy. In tetanic contractions(B), the total activity related heat when plotted as a function of tension-time integral is also depressed in PTU as compared to control. According to [27].*

Independent of the type of contraction (twitch or tetanic), the type of heat (total activity related heat = initial heat plus recovery heat), or the mechanical equivalent (peak tension or tension-time integral) significantly more heat was released per mechanical parameter in the control (αα) than in the hypothyrotic (PTU, ββ) myocardium. Figure 18 depicts similar data for pressure overload rat myocardium (GOP = Goldblatt). Changes of the composition of contractile protein expressed as percent β–myosin heavy chain have been shown to directly correlate with economy of contraction (Figure 19). An exponential function

may fit this relation better than a linear regression equation. Similar data were obtained for the pressure-overloaded rabbit myocardium [29] and the hypothyrotic rat myocardium by other authors [30].

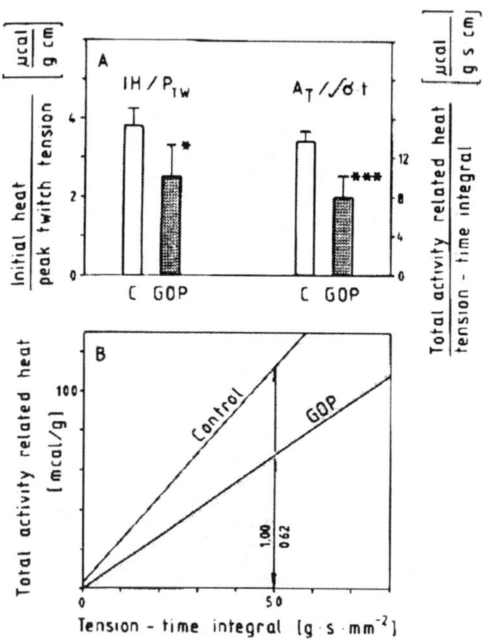

*Figure 18: Economy of myocardial contraction in hypertensive Goldblatt (GOP) rats in twitches (**A**) and tetanic contractions (**B**). Economy of twitches is analyzed by either relating initial heat to peak twitch tension (IH/P_{TW}) on the left or relating total activity-related heat to tension-time integral ($A_T/\int\sigma t$) on the rigt. Both indices decrease in GOP as compared to C (control) indicating a better economy. In tetanic contractions (B), the total activity-related heat when plotted as a function of tension-time integral is also depressed. According to [27].*

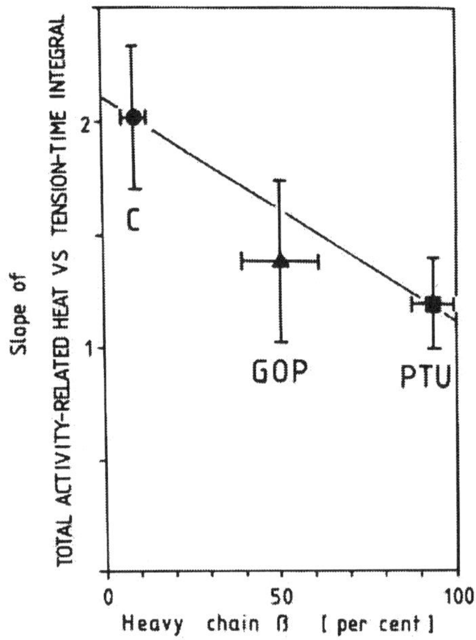

Figure 19: Relationship between the slope of total activity-related heat vs tension-time integral, which is an inverse measure of contraction economy (see Figures 17B and 18B), and the content of myosin heavy chain ß. The more myosin heavy chain ß, the lower the slope of the function, the better the economy of contraction. C, control; GOP, Goldblatt; PTU, propylthiouracil, i.e., hypothyrotic. According to [27].

4.3.3. Acute Changes of Energetics in Human Myocardium

Although many mechanical experimental studies have been performed worldwide regarding human myocardium and acute pharmacological interventions, to our knowledge there is only one report on myothermal measurements in human myocardium as it is influenced by acute pharmacological interventions. Hasenfuss and coworkers [31] compared the influence of isoproterenol and ouabain on human end-stage failing myocardium. As expected from animal cardiac muscle experiments, ouabain had only a relatively small but significant effect on tension-independent heat (+61 %) indicating somewhat more calcium ions being cycled during one twitch, whereas isoproterenol increased calcium-dependent heat release by 246 %. Therefore, regarding excitation-contraction coupling, ouabain is much more economical to stimulate failing human myocardium compared to β_1-adrenoceptor stimulation. However, Hasenfuss et al. did not find differences in the mechanics or energetics of cross-bridges when ouabain intervention is compared to isoproterenol application. These findings do neither agree with our results in animal studies (non-failing myocardium) nor with our data obtained by using the frequency-response method (see Chapter VI).These discrepancies may result from two different aspects: (1) In animal studies, non-failing myocardial tissues are used which *are* highly sensitive towards β_1-adrenoceptor stimulation. In failing myocardium, the response to isoproterenol is attenuated due to β-receptor downregulation and other subcellular adaptation mechanisms. (2) In the study of Hasenfuss et al., the ratio between tension-dependent heat and tension-time integral differs greatly between the two experimental sets (ouabain vs. isoproterenol). Therefore, the uneconomical effect of isoproterenol on the contractile proteins (cross-bridge cycling) may have been missed in this study.

4.3.4. Chronic Changes in Energetics of Human Myocardium

Initially, scientists doubted that human myocardium might have the same plasticity to adapt to pressure overload and hormonal alterations like the myocardium of small rodents. This view was based on the fact that in human ventricular myocardium one could find almost pure V3 isomyosin (ββ-homodimer). This was in contrast to atrial human myocardium, in which V1, V2, and V3 myosins are present, and changes of those have been demonstrated with mechanical consequences (Chapter III).

However, when analyzing the human left ventricular myocardium with respect to energetics using the myothermal method, it became clear that the human myocardium must have adaptive mechanisms on the level of the contractile proteins to alter the cross-bridge force-time integral. This has been shown for volume overload (mitral regurgitation) [32] and dilated cardiomyopathy [33]. Figure 20 shows the calculated cross-bridge force-time integral (for details in calculation procedure see section 3.A. of this chapter) plotted as a function of percent V3 myocardium for a variety of species and diseases [32]. Although human (both control and overload) myocardium exhibits 100 % V3, a significant increase in the cross-bridge force-time integral is observed in human overload. On the other hand, differences in force-time integral in rat and rabbit myocardium correlate well with the content of percent V3 myocardium. In human dilated cardiomyopathy, again, an increase in force-time integral was observed similar to human volume overload [33].

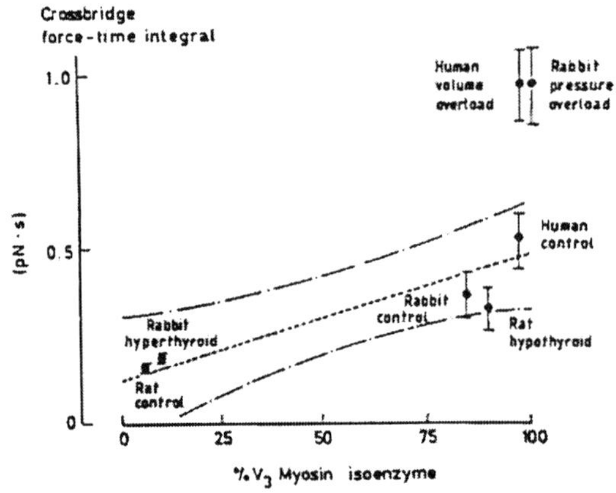

Figure 20: Relationship between crossbridge force-time integral and amount of V_3 myosin isoenzyme. In general, there is a linear relationship between the crossbridge force-time integral and the V_3 myosin isoenzyme. However, in the volume overloaded human myocardium and in the pressure overloaded rabbit myocardium there is an increase in crossbridge force-time integral despite almost pure V_3 myosin isoenzyme in the respective controls. According to [32].

The question, which arises from these data, regards the molecular basis which might explain these functional and energetic differences: Three different hypotheses have been suggested: (1) Isoforms of troponin T might be not only present, but rather responsible for these energetic differences [34]. (2) Composition and phosphorylation status of light chains may play a role [35,36]. (3) Very small content of α-isomyosin may play a role in human non-failing myocardium and might be absent in human overload and failing myocardium [37,38] (detailed discussion in chapter VI).

4.4. Discussion

The changes observed in the mammalian myocardium in the acute or chronic setting may be interpreted in two different ways:

(1) The slowing of the cross-bridge cycling rate combined with an increased force-time integral of a cross-bridge has been judged to be beneficial, because for a unit of force development (over time) less energy is needed, and therefore, the contraction process is economically improved from an energetic point of view.

(2) However, slowing contraction velocity has detrimental effects on the power output of a muscle system as demonstrated in Figure 21.

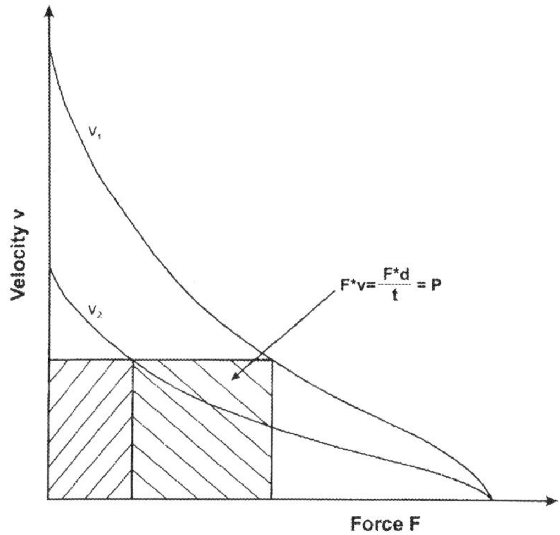

Figure 21: Schematic force-velocity relationships: V_1, fast cardiac muscle; V_2, slow cardiac muscle; V, velocity; F, force; d, distance; t, time; P, power. The cross-hatched areas indicate the different power of the two muscles

Provided the same strength of two muscles with different contraction velocities, the slower muscle has much less power than the fast muscle, because power is calculated as the product from velocity and force. Therefore, biological mechanisms that slow the contraction velocity increase economy and decrease power output, whereas catecholamines and related compounds reduce economy but increase power output (see also Figure 10 in Chapter VI).

REFERENCES

1) Gerthsen, Kneiser, Vogel: Physik: Ein Lehrbuch zum Gebrauch neben Vorlesungen. Springer-Verlag, Berlin, Heidelberg, New York 1977

2) Hill AV: The energy degraded in the recovery process of stimulated muscle. J Physiol 1913;46:28-80

3) Abbott BC: The heat production associated with the maintenance of a prolonged contraction and the extra heat produced during large shortening. J Physiol 1951;112:438-445

4) Gibbs CL: Cardiac energetics. Physiol Rev 1978;58:174-254

5) Mulieri LA, Luhr G, Trefry J, Alpert NR: Metal-film thermopiles for use with rabbit right ventricular papillary muscles. Am J Physiol 1977;233:C146-156

6) Hill AV, Woledge RC: An examination of absolute values in myothermic measurements. J Physiol (Lond) 1962;162:311-333

7) Kretschmer KM, Wilkie DR: A new method for absolute heat measurements utilizing the Peltier effect. J Physiol (Lond) 1972;224:18P-20P

8) Hamrell BB, Pannaanan R, Trono J, Alpert NR: A stable, sensitive, low-compliance force transducer. J Appl Physiol 1975;38:190-193

9) Frank O: Zur Dynamik des Herzmuskels. J Biol 1895;32:370-447. Translation from German: Chapman CP, Wasserman EB: On the dynamics of cardiac muscle. Am Heart J 1959;58:282-317

10) Starling EH: Linacre Lecture on the Law of the Heart. London, England; Longmans: 1918

11) Bowditch HP: Über die Eigentümlichkeiten der Reizbarkeit welche Muskelfasern des Herzens zeigen. Ber Sachs Ges Akkad 1871;23:652-689

12) Sarnoff SJ, Brockman SK, Gilmore JP, Linden RJ, Mitchell JH: Regulation of ventricular contraction: influence of cardiac sympathetic and vagal nerve stimulation on atrial and ventricular dynamics. Circ Res 1960;8:1108-1122

13) Holubarsch Ch, Pieske B, Kretschmann B, Schmidt-Schweda S, Meyer M, Schlotthauer K, Ruf T, Hasenfuss G, Just H: The functional role of angiotensin and endothelin in failing and nonfailing human myocardium. In: Dhalla NS, Beamish RE, Takeda N, Nagano M, eds. The Failing Heart. Philadelphia, PA: Lippincott-Raven;1995:295-304

14) Gibbs CL, Gibson WR: Effects of alterations in the stimulus rate upon energy output, tension development and tension-time integral of cardiac muscle in rabbits. Circ Res 1970;27:611-618

15) Alpert NR, Blanchard EM, Mulieri LA: Tension-independent heat in rabbit papillary muscle. J Physiol (Lond) 1989;414:433-453

16) Gwathmey JK, Hajjar RJ, Solaro RJ: Contractile deactivation and uncoupling of crossbridges. Circ Res 1991;69:1280-1292

17) Holubarsch Ch, Hasenfuss G, Just H, Alpert NR: Positive inotropism and myocardial energetics: influence of ß-receptor agonist stimulation, phosphodiesterase inhibition, and ouabain. Cardiovascular Res 1994;28:994-1002

18) Ruf T, Hebisch S, Groß R, Alpert NR, Just H, Holubarsch Ch: Modulation of myocardial economy and efficiency in mammalian failing and nonfailing myocardium by calcium channel activation and ß-adrenergic stimulation. Cardiovascular Res 1996;32:1047-1055

19) Holubarsch Ch: New inotropic concepts: Rationale for and differences between calcium sensitizers and phosphodiesterase inhibitors. Cardiology 1997;88(Suppl 2):12-20

20) Alpert NR, Hamrell BB, Halpen W: Mechanical and biochemical correlates of cardiac hypertrophy. Circ Res 1974;34/35(Suppl II):71-82

21) Jacob R, Ebrecht G, Kämmereit A, Medugorac I, Wendt-Gallitelli MF: Myocardial function in different models of cardiac hypertrophy. An attempt of correlating mechanical, biochemical and morphological parameters. Basic Res Cardiol 1977;72:160-166

22) Yazaki Y, Raben MS: Effect of the thyroid state on the enzymatic characteristics of cardiac myosin. A difference in behavior of rat and rabbit cardiac myosin. Circ Res 1975;36:208-215

23) Lompré AM, Schwartz K, d'Albis A, Lacombe G, Van Thiem N, Swynghedauw B: Myosin isoenzyme redistribution in chronic heart overload. Nature 1979;282:105-107

24) Hoh JFY, McGrath PA, Hale PT: Electrophoretic analysis of multiple form of rat cardiac myosin. Effects of hypophysectomy and thyrosine replacement. J Mol Cell Cardiol 1977;10:1053-1076

25) Dillmann WH: Diabetes mellitus and hypothyroidism induce changes in myosin distribution in the rat heart – do alterations in fuel flux mediate these changes? Adv Exp Med Biol 1986;194:469-479

26) Holubarsch Ch, Goulette R, Mulieri LA, Alpert NR: Heat liberation in experimentally induced tetanic contractions of myocardium from normal and Goldblatt rats. Cardiac adaption to hemodynamic overload, training and stress. Dr. Steinkopff Verlag 1983:158-166

27) Holubarsch Ch, Litten RZ, Mulieri LA, Alpert NR: Energetic changes of myocardium as an adaptation to chronic hemodynamic overload and thyroid gland activity. Bas Res Cardiol 1985;80:582-593

28) Holubarsch Ch, Goulette RP, Litten RZ, Martin BJ, Mulieri LA, Alpert NR: The economy of isometric force development, myosin isoenzyme pattern and myofibrillar ATPase activity in normal and hypothyroid rat myocardium. Circ Res 1985;56:78-86

29) Alpert NR, Mulieri LA: Increased myothermal economy of isometric force generation in compensated cardiac hypertrophy induced by pulmonary artery constriction in rabbit. A characterization of heat liberation in normal and hypertrophied right ventricular papillary muscles. Circ Res 1982;50:491-500

30) Loiselle DS, Wendt IR, Hoh JFY: Energetic consequences of thyroid-modulated shifts in ventricular isomyosin distribution in the rat. J Muscle Res Cell Motil 1982;3:5-23

31) Hasenfuss G, Mulieri LA, Allen PD, Just H, Alpert NR: Influence of isoproterenol and ouabain on excitation-contraction coupling, crossbridge function, and energetics in failing human myocardium. Circulation 1996;94:3155-3160

32) Hasenfuss G, Mulieri LA, Blanchard EM, Holubarsch Ch, Leavitt BJ, Ittleman F, Alpert NR: Energetics of isometric force development in control- and volume-overload human myocardium. Comparison with animal species. Circ Res 1991;68:836-846

33) Hasenfuss G, Mulieri LA, Leavitt BJ, Allen PD, Haeberle JR, Alpert NR: Alteration of contractile function and excitation-contraction coupling in dilated cardiac myopathy. Circ Res 1992;70:1225-1232

34) Anderson PAW, Malouf NN, Oakeley AE, Pagani ED, Allen PD: Troponin T isoform expression in humans. A comparison among normal and failing adult heart, fetal heart, and adult and fetal skeletal muscle. Circ Res 1991;69:1226-1233

35) Hirzel HO, Tuchschmid CR, Schneider J, Krayenbuehl HP, Schaub MC: Relationship between myosin isoenzyme composition, hemodynamics, and myocardial structure in various forms of human cardiac hypertrophy. Circulation Research 1985;57:729-40

36) Morano I: Effects of different expression and posttranslational modifications of myosin light chains on contractility of skinned human cardiac fibers. Basic Res Cardiol 1992;87(Suppl I):129-141

37) Lowes Bd, Minobe W, Abraham WT, et al.: Changes in gene expression in the intact human heart. Downregulation of α-myosin heavy chain in hypertrophied, failing ventricular myocardium. J Clin Invest 1997;100:2315-2324

38) Nakao K, Minobe W, Roden R, Bristow WR, Leinwand LA: Myosin heavy chain gene expression in human heart failure. J Clin Invest 1997;100:2370-2372

5. SKINNED CARDIAC FIBRES

5.1. Introduction

The pumping action of the heart is the driving force of the cardiovascular system that supplies all organs and tissues with blood. The mechanical basis behind generation of sufficient pressure for this task lies in the ability of the myocyte to shorten. Shortening is a process mainly determined by the interaction of myosin and actin. They are the motor proteins of the muscular tissue. The acto-myosin interaction, which forms cross-bridge cycling, is the basic mechanism that underlies generation of force. The regulation of kinetics of that acto-myosin interaction has, therefore, profound impact on the performance of the heart [1,2,3].

Calcium is a key regulator of myocardial contraction. When the intracellular calcium concentration rises after excitation, calcium binds to its regulatory site on troponin C. The following recruitment of cross-bridges is able to develop force [4]. Three basic mechanisms regulate the contractile strength of the heart in the acute setting. First, muscle force and stroke volume vary directly with sarcomere length and preload, respectively, phenomena broadly referred to as the Frank-Starling law of the heart. Second, myocardial force development is heart rate dependent; peak isometric force increases with heart rate in normal mammalian myocardium, including human cardiac muscle. Third, cardiac muscle is under neurohormonal control, including the sympathetic and vagal nervous system and some polypeptides such as angiotensin and endothelin. The long term changes involve by either physiological or pathological demand the alteration of intracellular components, which are associated with changes in biochemistry and function [5,6].

In heart disease, with respects to hypertrophy and congestive heart failure, mainly alterations of calcium handling have been evidenced. In addition, there are indications for structural changes of the contractile apparatus and altered regulatory mechanisms [7]. It is of major clinical importance to know about these alterations, since heart failure is an often seen clinical syndrome [8]. A pharmacological intervention can mainly be improved on the basis of understanding the pathophysiological mechanisms. In the treatment of heart failure it is the ultimate wish to find positive inotropic substances, which have no, or even negative, chronotropic effects, should not be mediated by increases in calcium transients, and should decelerate, rather than accelerate, cross-bridge kinetics. This was expected from the so-called calcium sensitizers. The principles of the therapy in congestive heart failure are based on an improvement of the economy of the heart by decreasing heart rate, wall tension and cross-bridge cycling [9,10].

To investigate muscular mechanics and energetics regarding heart action and its regulatory mechanisms many physiological methods have been developed [11,12]. In this chapter, special interest is focused on the skinned fibre method. Since an isolated multicellular preparation extensively demembranated can neither be stimulated electrically nor produce adenosine triphosphate [13], research in concern to the excitation-contraction coupling is rather impossible. Skinned fibres are not able to contract after an action potential. We will have a closer look onto calcium, sarcomere length and neurohormonal regulation processes in terms of cross-bridge cycling. It is the special feature of the skinned fibre method to investigate mechanisms that underlie the interaction of the contractile proteins and direct influences on these [14].

5.2. Methods

The skinning of muscle fibres offers the possibility to investigate direct effects on the contractile apparatus without the influence of various structural and mechanical constraints [11].

As we understand the mechanism of the process that we call „skinning", at first a fiber is prepared out of the trabecular structure of the muscle and the endocardium when experiments are done with heart muscle. Afterwards the cell's membrane is permeabilized or totally taken apart. Different methods are optional to use with different effects. Dependant on the last step, the sarcolemma's fatty acids and even those of other membrane holding structures like mitochondria and sarcoplasmic reticulum (SR) are solubilized chemically or mechanically disrupted (Figure 1). This evokes that the membrane becomes more permeable for larger structural units. During the skinning process, proteins by permeability and fatty acids by dissolution leave the cell and lack in their function. The consequence is a sincere, destructive influence on the membrane's stability, the cell's homeostasis and furthermore the cell's signalling systems (Figure 1).

An extensively skinned fibre can neither be stimulated nor produce ATP [13]. Thus a skinned fibre is either in a state of relaxation or calcium contracture. The surrounding solution has direct influence on the contractile proteins because intracellular and extracellular solution media are of identical composition. This composition of the solution has to be chosen by the experimenting person. We define activating and relaxing solutions for the experiment – see below.

5.2.1. The Process of Skinning

In case of chemical skinning, we define special solutions. The solution for solubilization of membranes is called a skinning solution. The process of chemically skinning includes the dissolution of the cell membrane and intracellular, membranous structures.

Substances being used for this purpose are triton X-100, saponin and lubrol WX [13,15,16]. Quite recently streptolysin O has been described for skinning by Fawcett et al. [17]. The concentration of Triton X-100 is about 1 Vol. % [13]. Saponin has been used at concentrations of 50 µg/ml up to 250 µg/ml [18]. Besides the skinning solution experimental success is greatly dependent on the preparation of the muscle, including the removement of the endothelium. Last but not least, the time of induration is essential for the quality of the experiment. The time determines the chemical skinning as a main factor dependent on the diameter of the fiber, the type of tissue used - whether it is animal or human, skeletal or cardiac muscle tissue - , and the methodical setup. A difference from 0.5 to 12 hours has been reported [19,20]. It should be noted that based on our own experience the skinning procedure of failing human myocardium takes longer time, since alterations as fibrosis have impact on its handling in this concern. Additionally, glycerol extraction is done by using 50%Vol. glycerol as soluble mean [21].

For ventricular heart muscle, the mechanical skinning has not had a real break-through. The more difficult preparation of the short muscle cells may be one reason (<50µm) [22]. Another opportunity in skinning offers the way of freezing the trabecles in liquid N_2 resulting in less extensive loss of force during the experiment [23]. Podolsky [24] described the mechanical skinning in a relaxing solution or paraffin oil.

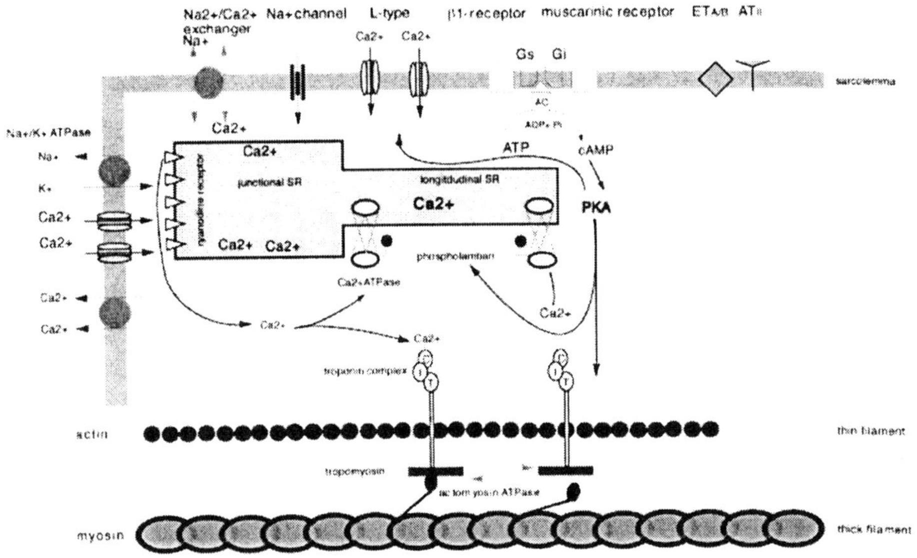

Figure 1: Scheme of a cardiac muscle cell and important signaling pathways: Structures that are destroyed or at least influenced by skinning procedeures are the cell membrane including its channels, tranport systems and receptors with dependent signalling systems and the sarcoplasmic reticulum including the ryanodine receptors and calcium ATPases.

5.2.2. Storing The Fibre

Even more these fibres can be stored at about –20 °C for a certain time in a so-called storing solution. In our studies, apart from the detergent, the storing solution consists of the same chemical substances as the relaxing solution. The used solvent is aqua bidest and glycerol in equal volumes [21]. The time of possible storing depends on the special experimental conditions. The more sensitive these conditions are, namely ATPase activity measurement and sarcomere length detection, the shorter the time of storing must be chosen. A storing up to one month has been described for successful experiments. It shall be emphasized, however, that the immediate use is the best [25,26,27].

Besides time also temperature has great influence on the quality of the fibre. Above 0°C a decrease in force of more than 50 % has to be expected. Exposure to warmth should be avoided for reproducibility. To store the fibers at –20°C seems to be sufficient. The main advantage of storing human myocardium is the independence of the heart transplantation frequency.

5.2.3. Activating and Relaxing Solutions

The composition of activating and relaxing solutions is essential for skinned fibre experiments. The aim is to create solutions similar to the intracellular liquid. The proposed content and experimental constellation bring about to compromise, because a number of other necessary substances has to be added. Some of these are highly concentrated chelators, buffers, ATP regenerating systems and enzymes [28].

As mentioned above the main difference between an activating and a relaxing solution is the free calcium concentration [29]. Fabiato and Fabiato [30] created the basics of software that were important to develop solutions used today. The basics for the used solutions have been provided mainly on their experiences as well as of those from Godt and Lindley [31]. Thus, differentiated ionic buffer systems can be created: Free sarcoplasmatic calcium is about 0.1 µM to 0.1 mM. Evident values for free magnesium concentration are 0.1 to 3 mM. Magnesium mostly binds to adenosinetriphosphate. MgATP complex is reported to exist in concentrations from 3 to 5 mM. Furthermore, monovalent cations as potassium and sodium ions and monovalent anions like chloride ions belong to these systems. The physiological ionic strength is supposed to be at about 0.15 to 0.25. Almost ever the described pH is fixed at 7.00. In respect to temperature conditions, mostly room temperature is chosen although a lower temperature is reported to significantly reduce muscle destroying mechanisms during the experiment [32,31]. It is demanded to control temperature as well as all other parameters. Overestimation of the purity of EGTA which is used as the main calcium buffering compound in the relaxing and activating solutions for skinned fibre experiments [29] has been calculated to accumulate in a more than 3-fold over- or underestimation of the calculated free Ca^{2+}-concentration (by 0.5 pCa units) [33,34].

For creating solutions, we used the software developed by Güth (Scientific Instruments, Heidelberg). Important to know is that herewith an about 10% lower potassium concentration is demanded. This affects the force-calcium relation (see below) of the muscle fibre in a rightward shift. Induced maximum force could be reduced [35,36,37].

A pCa of 7.0 to 9.0 doesn't activate a skinned fibre [38]. pCa is defined as the negative decadic logarithm of free calcium concentration. A solution with a calcium concentration ranging from calcium free to pCa 4 does not exist under physiological conditions. A controlled continuous process in occupying calcium binding regulatory sites of contractile proteins is possible ending in a complete calcium activation [39,40]. Threshold Ca^{2+}-concentrations (denoting the minimum calcium concentration needed to evoke a contractile response) have been reported in the range of pCa 5.9 to 7.3 [40,41,42]. Great impact on this more than 10-fold difference in values has the specific composition of the buffered solutions, which leads to inaccuracies in the calculation of the free calcium concentration. Note that unphysiologically high calcium concentrations destroy the fibre to be shown in a rapid loss in generated force after steady state [42,43].

On the whole, we also have to consider pharmacological and physiological aspects chosen with the experiment as well as differences between species.

When discussing necessary substances for the solutions, we did mention about substances that are chosen only by some research groups dependant on their experiences. Those are for instance sodium azide (NaN_3), oligomycin B, A2P5, creatine phosphate (CP) or creatine phosphokinase (CPK). The use of NaN_3 bases on an additional effect in chemical skinning which results in the destruction of ATP-dependent membrane proteins [44]. The inhibition of bacterial growth and thus of bacterial ATP consumption is another effect that is as well supported by oligomycin B and A2P5 [19]. CP and CPK together form an ATP regenerating system used to prevent a lack of ATP deeply inside the fibre that is likely to occur [46].

5.2.4. Activating a Skinned Fibre

During activation a fibre develops force. Force per cross sectional area is defined as tension. It is to differentiate between tension during relaxation, i.e., resting tension [47b], and active tension developed during activation. The sum of both we call total tension. Absolute force divided by maximum force describes relative force that is expressed in % or values from 0 to 1.

The basic protocol on skinned fibre experiments includes attachment of the skinned fibre preparation to force transducer and linear motor at slack length, stretch for optimal sarcomere length, relaxation in pCa 8 solution and activation with pCa 4 to maximum force. The latter step should be done for reasons of reproducibility at least one time before the actual measurement. When increasing pCa, tension under steady-state conditions has to be waited for. Skinned fibre experiments investigate comparisons of a number of activations (at least two) under isometric steady state conditions.

5.2.5. Skinning procedure – a historical approach

Mechanical skinning has been performed by stripping muscle fibres in relaxing solution or paraffin oil. The muscle cell membrane and a superficial layer of myofibrils can be teased off with sharp steel needles [24]. The method of mechanical skinning was introduced by Natori in 1954 using skeletal muscle [47a]. Equivalent preparations of cardiac muscle cells are described by Fabiato in 1982 who had to modify this technique since cardiac cells are much shorter in size [48]. Especially this type of skinning without removal of the sarcoplasmic reticulum allows to study its function mainly investigated by Fabiato and Fabiato [49,50,51]. Stienen and co-workers have given a description of a freeze-drying method which shall be mentioned here [23].

Chemical skinning. It is possible to imagine that a chemical skinning procedure is easier to handle in respect to the preparation. Glycerol extraction as a chemical process of permeabilization [53] was used systematically at first by Weber and Portzehl [54]. Their aim was to remove all the intrinsic ATP from skeletal muscle fibres by making the cell membrane highly permeable to ATP with aqueous glycerol solutions. Nayler and Merrillees [21] described a similar proceeding and compared glycerinated and intact muscle preparation in their differences. Later on Schädler in 1967 considered skinned fiber experiments with cardiac muscle as an important tool to compare differences in muscular tissue [55]. Solaro et al. in 1971 performed fundamental research on skinning by using the detergent Triton-X 100 in canine heart muscle [13]. With this chemical substance a removal of all membrane structures is possible including the sarcolemma, as well as the sarcoplasmic reticulum and the mitochondria. Triton X-100 gave a breakthrough for skinned fiber research and has been used mainly and widely. Saponin is a detergent that induces hyperpermeability. Just alike mechanical skinning the substance does not induce any destruction of intracellular lipid membranes. This gives the chance to control the cells function without affection of intracellular structures as compared to Triton-X 100. Above all, for investigastion of the sarcoplasmic reticulum saponin offered great perspectives [56,15].

The approach to investigate human cardiac muscle by using the skinned fiber technique happened in the late eigthies. Questions regarding species differences as well as pathological states (hypertrophied and failing) were addressed [27,57]. Latest news report from preparations of myotubes which were permeabilized after generation in transfected quail myoblasts to research mutants of cardiac troponin T (TnT) [58]. Very recently, Streptolysin O has been reported to be another substance postulated to work for skinning [17].

5.2.6. Ca^{2+}-Force Relationships

Concerning the relation between free Ca^{2+}-concentration and developed force of a single muscle preparation the named method is a gold standard in physiological muscle experiments [44,58b,36].

To detect isometric force the skinned trabeculum has to be fixed at one end to a force transducer element [59,60]. For isometric tension measurement the other end has to be stationary. For fixing the fibre, aluminium clips, glue, nylon snares and metal tweezers are described [60,61,62,63]. In case of quick-release, shortening or oszillation experiments the latter end has to be fixed to a linear motor, also called displacement generator [18,6].

The establishment of high Ca^{2+}-concentration in a step-like rapid manner is quite difficult, because the Ca^{2+} diffusion is quite slow. For a long time, the activation of the muscle fiber was only possible by an exchange of the solutions containing different Ca^{2+}-concentrations. First improvements were achieved by introducing the Ca^{2+} jump technique [64]. Thereby, an increase in Ca^{2+} is possible within 0.2 sec. This is almost as fast as in living muscle fibers [65]. These fast switches were necessary to set a highly concentrated buffer solution for to stabilize highly Ca^{2+}-concentration containing solutions. Since the use of buffers developed for clamping ionized Ca^{2+}, there is no need for anymore [66,30]. For skinned fibres, the usage of single activation solutions with different calcium concentrations is one way, another one is the gradient method realized by Güth. The latter describes the constant mixture of just two solutions, a relaxing (pCa 8) and an activating solution (pCa 4). The fiber is activated step by step when simultaneously a determined volume of pCa 4 solution is added to the afferent part of the system containing relaxing solution. A constant calcium concentration acceleration evokes a steady increase in activation. The aim is not to look on one single status of activation but the complete process. More detailed curves are received. But both ways keep advantages and disadvantages (see Figure 2).

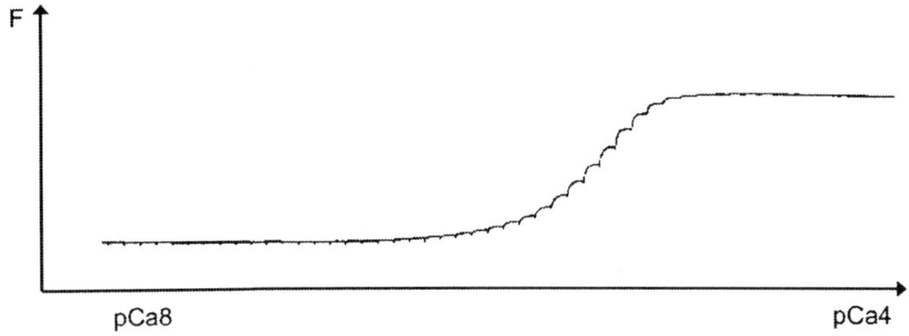

Figure 2: Activation of a skinned human cardiac fibre. Force increases with increasing Ca^{2+}-concentration induced by steady increase of Ca^{2+} in the gradient mixing procedure (original data).

5.2.7. Control of Sarcomere Length

The sarcomere as a basic repetitive structure unit in muscle tissue is able to shorten through sliding filaments [67]. To picture muscle cells in such detail electron microscopy offers an elegant way. Apart from the contractile apparatus also capillaries, intercalated disks, mitochondria and stroma can easily be differentiated. A great approach on the ultrastructure of cardiac muscle was done by Fawcett and McNutt [68] (for further review see [4,11]).

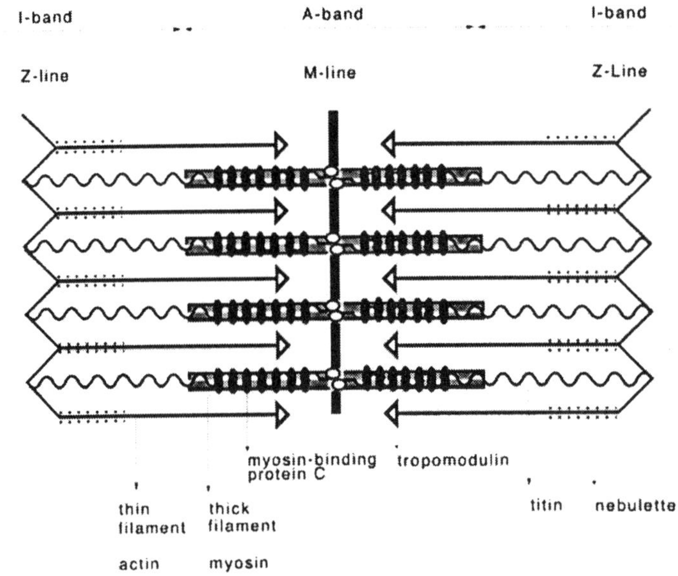

Figure 3: The structure of the sarcomere and its relating appearance in optical microscopy. Modified according to [69].

However, to measure simultaneously both muscle function, i.e., force development and possibly shortening, and sarcomere length, the contractile proteins have to remain functionally intact during the process of sarcomere length measurements. This has been first achieved by X-ray diffraction studies [70] and later on by optical diffraction [71].

Considering the muscle preparation as an optic lattice, the laws of optic diffraction can be applied. If monochromatic light (laser) is directed vertically against a single slit, diffraction of the light waves occurs: Giving a certain angle α, the distance CB equals the length of the light wave, and the distance DE equals half of the light wave length.

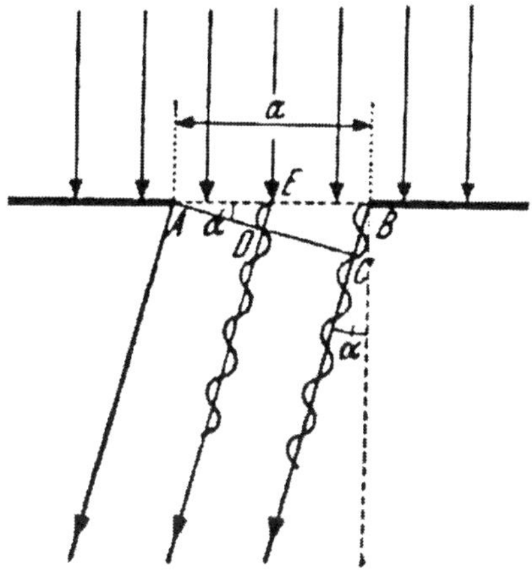

Figure 4: Optical diffraction explained on the basis of a single slit with the width a

As a consequence the light beam through the points *E* and *D* is dissolved by the beam through the points *BC* due to interference. In other words, if the distance *CB* equals the light wave length or is a multiplication product of it, dissolution of the light occurs (diffraction minimum) due to the following equation (see also Figure 4):

$a \cdot \sin\alpha = n \cdot \lambda$,

when $n = 1,2,3,4...$ (whole numbers)

a = width of the single slit

α = angle of the diffracted beam

λ = wave length of the laser beam

The function of intensity (*I*) of the light is given by

$I = [\sin^2(\pi \cdot (a/\lambda) \cdot \sin\alpha] / [(\sin\alpha)^2]$.

In a muscle preparation, there is no single slit but rather the intensity maxima of the single slit infer with each other depending on the distance between the slits. This distance is called the lattice constant d (or δ).

In analogy to the single slit experiment, the intensity maximum is given as follows:

$\delta \cdot \sin\alpha = n \cdot \lambda$.

The function of intensity I of the vertically directed and diffracted light is determined by the following function:

$I = [[\sin^2(\pi \cdot (\alpha/\lambda) \cdot \sin\alpha)] / [(\sin\alpha)^2]] \cdot [\cos^2(\pi \cdot \delta \cdot \sin\alpha/\lambda)]$.

The very strong central light beam (a = 0°) is called the maximum of zero degree. For the maximum of the first degree, which is relevant for sarcomere length measurement, the following equation is valid using a laser beam of 670 nm:

$$\text{sarcomere length } (\mu m) = 0.670\ \mu m / \sin \alpha .$$

Based on the above described theory, sarcomeric structures of the muscle can be analyzed on a paper screen by the naked eye [72]. The following rule has to be considered: The greater the number of slits, the sharper the maxima; however, the fibre preparation has to be sufficiently thin to allow the light transmission through it [73].

5.2.8. ATPase Activity Measurement

Adenosine triphosphate (ATP), in general, is mainly used as an energy source by the myofilaments (tension generation and cell shortening), for intracellular calcium handling, and for maintaining the intracellular milieu through ATP dependent ion transports. The investigation of energetic aspects of muscle contraction by Fenn [74,75] was just the beginning for other methods being developed to determine energy consumption: Measurements of heat production [74,75,76,77,36] and oxygen consumption provide indirect methods to measure ATPase activity. Whereas for skinned fibres indirect measurement was possible by Edman's observations [78], at first, more recently reported methods allow a direct measurement in terms of ATP hydrolysis rate [60,79].

Several constellations of methods and instruments are described for the detection of ATPase activity of which the most important will shortly be described in the following.

(1) ATPase activity measurements on the basis of the so-called laser photolysis method [79]. Goldman et al. [79] described a new method "for studying the reaction kinetics of the force-generating mechanism in muscle". Here, inert photolabile precursors of ATP or adenosine diphosphate (ADP) are incorporated in skinned muscle fibres from rabbit psoas muscle. Then, laser pulse hydrolysis rapidly liberates the nucleotide. Thus, the resolution set by diffusion of nucleotide from the bathing medium is prevented. These measurements were done under rigor conditions. A solution which does not contain ATP brings the muscle fiber into rigor state [80]. Thereafter, caged ATP, the inert precursor of ATP, added to the bathing solution diffuses into the fibre. The application of a pulse of UV radiation from a frequency–doubled ruby laser initiates the photolysis of ATP to ADP and inorganic phosphate (P_i). Conditions of the laser

reached through frequency-doubling are a 150-mJ, 50-ns pulse of light at a wavelength of 347 nm. The photolysis solution was kept for ATP-assay reason using luciferin-luciferase after the fibre reached its relaxing status.

(2) ATPase activity measurements on the basis of an enzymatic-coupled assay using the Embden-Mayerhof-pathway's last steps in aerobic and anaerobic energy production (see Figure 5). [60,19,81].

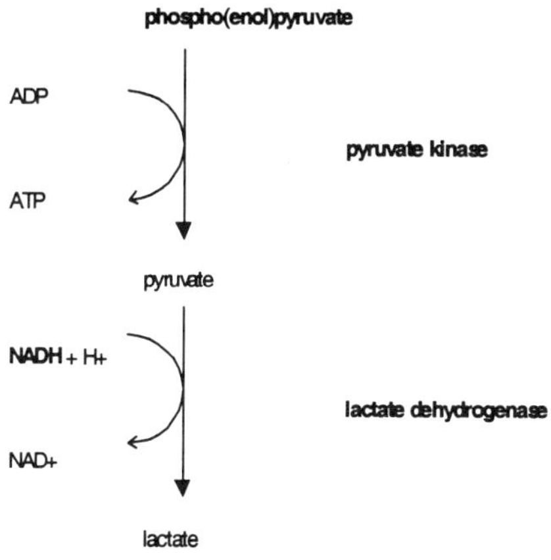

Figure 5: Biochemical basis of the detection of ATPase activity through fluorescence changes. Substances added to the experimental solution are set in heavy letters.

At the end of the aerobic glycolytic pathway the biochemical synthesis of pyruvate produces ATP, in addition. The equivalent enzyme to catalyze this reaction is pyruvate kinase. Further synthesis of lactate under anaerobic conditions includes the oxidization of NADH + H^+ to NAD^+, a reaction that is catalyzed by lactate dehydrogenase. The point of interest is that NADH fluoresces at 470nm, in excited state at 340nm and NAD^+ does not. The consumption of ATP which urges the cascade to go on with the breakdown of NADH + H^+ to NAD^+ enables to detect ATPase activity by the photometrical determination of NADH's absorbance of UV light. Between ATP and NADH there is aequimolar condition (see Figure 5). Important to note that only a small range of NADH concentrations can be used to receive reliable ATPase activity determinations.

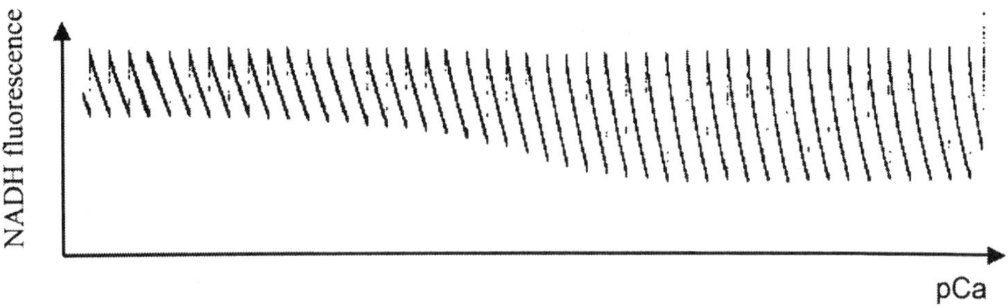

Figure 6: Example of ATPase activity measurement by detection of the decreasing fluorescent signal of NADH. By increasing calcium concentration (abszissa), acto-myosin ATPase is stimulated. Therefore, NADH fluorescence decreases with proportional increase in consumption of ATP (solution is triggered in the gradient mixture).

Important to know for the interpretation of NADH's fluorescence in the relaxing state of the fibre is to have the following things in mind: (1) photo bleaching: light not generated by the illumination system can also cause oxidization of NADH + H^+ to NAD^+; (2) ADP-contamination of enzymes; (3) non-specific ATPases not sufficiently inhibited; and (4) bacteria. This background signal has to be held as low as possible. In concern to human heart we would like to point out that it can not be expected to reach as low background fluorescence as in animal measurements. The light is produced by a special xenon high pressure lamp projecting its light through the bath. The fluorescent signal sent out by NADH is detected by a photometer (see Figure 5).

We want to mention as well DANZ-labeled Ca^{2+} transient measurements which have its special use in the functional understanding of TnC, since TnCDANZ fluorescence indicates Ca^{2+}-binding to the Ca^{2+}-specific sites of TnCDANZ and attachment of cross-bridges to the actin filament [82,83].

5.3. Results

We will look on special approaches in skinned fiber research related to mechanical and energetic aspects of muscular tissues, especially heart muscle

5.3.1. Cross-Bridge Cycling

Force production is defind as unitary force per cross-bridge cycle. Velocity of displacement reflects kinetics. Force production and velocity of displacement mirror the influence of motor proteins in respects to contractility. A cross-bridge cycle develops through a series of successive conformational changes in the myosin head domain. The structural and mechanical changes in the cross bridge cycle are coupled to highly energetic, chemical reactions involving the hydrolysis of ATP to ADP and inorganic phosphate (P_i) [3]. Regarding the interaction of actin and myosin with ATP and its hydrolytic products, different affinity states result between these two contractile proteins. The main states can be dichotomicly devided into weakly binding and strongly binding cross-bridges. Weakly binding cross-bridges exhibit low affinity, do not produce force and oscillate rapidly between attached and detached states. As one might assume their stiffness is not of significant resistance to stretch. The dissociation of P_i and thus a shift from weakly binding cross-bridges to strongly binding cross-bridges is thought to be coupled with force production [84,85]. Resulting in an increased stiffness to passive stretch, strongly binding cross-bridges exhibit slower oscillations and correlate with a strong affinity of myosin to actin. The nucleotide-free state after release of ADP finishes a whole cross-bridge cycle. Rigor mortis shows the result in a fixed situation. The binding of a new ATP-substrate brings the cycle to start again (see Figure 7).

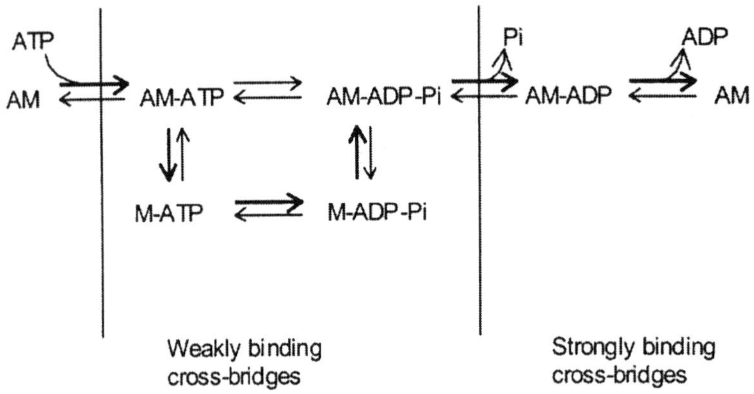

Figure 7: Simplified kinetic scheme of the cross-bridge cycle [69]. M, Myosin, A, Actin, Heavy arrows indicate main pathways. For explanations see text.

How to get information about the distribution of cross-bridges among weakly and strongly binding states and the kinetics of transitions between them? Measurements of contractile parameters such as isometric tension, shortening velocity and force redevelopment following a brief period of shortening at zero load give information.

In general, V_{max} (maximum shortening velocity) is roughly proportional to the ATPase activity and speed of contraction in heart as well as in skeletal muscles [78]. In the first quantitative model relating experimental parameters to the kinetics of the cross-bridge cycle two states were assumed: one attached and force-generating state and one detached and non-force-generating state [80]. Based on this model two equivalent rate constants of interaction are definded: the forward rate constant f determining the rate of attachment, and the forward rate constant g determining the rate of detachment. In the meantime, the model has undergone further developments resulting in many intermediate states of the acto-myosin fibrils during this chemical reaction [1,3]. But the original idea still forms the basis of theory. In analogy, the rate constant f_{app} describes the transition from weakly binding, non-force generating states, to the strongly binding, force generating state. Vice versa, g_{app} describes this event for the opposite transition via product release and rebinding of ATP (see Figure 7). The idea of attachment and detachment has been left, since weakly binding cross-bridges are known to be still in rapid equilibrium with actin. The following equation describes isometric force F for these conditions:

$F = F' \cdot n_{tot} \cdot f_{app} / (f_{app} + g_{app})$

F' is the force generated per cross-bridge cycle (unitary force).
n_{tot} is the total amount of cycling cross-bridges per half-saromere.
$f_{app} / (f_{app} + g_{app})$ equals the fraction of cross-bridges in force generating states and thus defines steady-state tension.

Either an increase in f_{app} or a decrease in g_{app} leads to an increase of the force generating cross-bridge fraction and finally results in an increased tension generation of a muscle. The rate of tension development after a brief shortening at zero load serves for the estimation of the rate of transitions from weakly to strongly binding states [3,86]. The rate constant of tension redevelopment (k_{td}) equals ($f_{app} + g_{app}$). The maximal shortening velocity, V_{max}, or ATPase activity, in general, primarily depends on g_{app} which, in turn, is controlled by the release of ADP [85]. During steady-state tension ATPase activity can be described by the following equation:

$ATPase = n_{tot} \cdot s \cdot f_{app} \cdot g_{app} / (f_{app} + g_{app})$

s is the number of half sarcomeres.

The division of the ATPase-equation by the force-equation yields the quotient
$g_{app} * s / F'$ showing the so-called tension cost.

Assuming isometric steady-state conditions s can be considered as a constant parameter. If *F'* is equal between two myosin isoforms under consideration, in addition, the relation of ATPase activity and tension may be directly proportional to g_{app}. Thus, an increase in g_{app} indicates an increase in tension cost, or a decrease in economy of force generation.

5.3.2. Calcium-Force Relationships

Concerning the relation between free Ca^{2+}-concentration and actively developed force of a single muscle the skinned fiber method is a gold standard. As we know, contractility is dependent on the contractile proteins on the one hand and on the intracellular Ca^{2+}-concentration on the other [87].

A special feature of heart muscle is that neither it contracts maximally during systole, nor it necessarily relaxes completely during diastole [88,89].

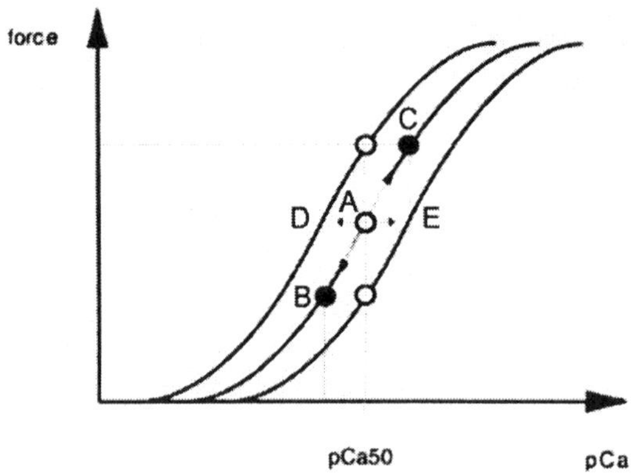

Figure 8: The Ca^{2+}-force relationship. Relative force is plotted versus negative decadic logarithm of increasing free Ca^{2+}-concentrations. pCa=negative decadic logarithm of free Ca^{2+}-ion concentration.

1) Increasing Ca^{2+} from A to C increases force proportional without affecting the Ca^{2+}-sensitivity (filled circles on the same curve).

2) At a given Ca^{2+}-concentration (open circles), force can be increased by increasing the Ca^{2+}-sensitivity of the contractile system (leftward shift; D), or lowered by decreasing Ca^{2+}-sensitivity (rightward shift; E).

3) The steepness of the pCa- force curve is a measure for the cooperativity of the activation process (Hill coefficient) and is unchanged in the given example.

According to [69].

To show how Ca^{2+} affects tension is expressed in the pCa-force relationship. In skinned fiber experiments, results are based on determinations under isometric steady-state conditions. Figure 8 schematically demonstrates typical pCa-force relationships: (1) The pCa_{50} indicates half maximal force. (2) Calcium sensitivity is increased when the curve is shifted to the left and decreased when shifted to the right. (3) The steepness of the curve is a measure of cooperativity: The normalized pCa-force data can be fitted to the Hill equation [90]:

HILL equation:

$$\text{fractional force } Y = \frac{[Ca2+]^{H}}{pCa_{50} + [Ca2+]^{H}}$$

Y names the fractional force, pCa_{50} the Ca^{2+}-concentration at half-maximal activation, which is an index for the affinity of Ca^{2+} to the contractile system. *H*, the so-called Hill coefficient, provides an index for cooperativity reflecting the minimal number of cooperating binding sites [91]

Regarding the correlation of free Ca^{2+}-force development in skinned preparations and intact muscles there are no clear findings. Whereas some groups have shown an agreement in this concern [38,92], others differ largely [93]. More recent data from skinned rat ventricular myocardium clearly support the latter ones [89]. On the other hand, this has not been confirmed in experiments with human ventricular muscle from failing and non-failing hearts [94]. The specific reasons have still not been proved. Harrison et al. [95] assumed that the lack of intracellular substances through skinning like carnosine and other buffering systems which significantly increase myofilament Ca^{2+}-sensitivity could play a role. In skinned preparations, the free Ca^{2+}-concentration was adjusted with Ca^{2+}-buffers (see above).

Fabiato [96] noticed that intact fiber preparations of vertebrate heart muscle never reached maximal force even under positiv inotropic intervention. At the same time, mean absolute force was about twice as high after skinning of the same preparations. The suggestion that the heart never works on a level more than half-maximal activation is close. Thus the heart has got reserves in variation of force by little decreases and increases in intracellular Ca^{2+}-concentration. In comparison, intact skeletal muscle is maximally activated at pCa 5. Here, small changes in intracellular and extracellular Ca^{2+} do not have influence on force development. That correlates with the finding that the heart does neither contract maximally during systole nor entirely relax during diastole [11].

Changes in the sensitivity of the contractile apparatus to Ca^{2+} may allow changes in force development. Compared to a shift to the right or left of the pCa-tension curve, at a certain Ca^{2+}-concentration the degree of activation changes, respectively. In terms of cross-bridge theory, increased numbers of acto-myosin interactions are hypothesized to enhance calcium sensitivity (cross-bridge induced calcium sensitivity increase) [97] or increase the rate of cross-bridge formation itself [98]. Ca^{2+}-sensitivity effects the pCa_{50}-value and the treshold Ca^{2+}-concentration. Concerning the pCa_{50}-values of mammalian heart muscle reports differ from 4.7-6.0 and 5.9-7.0, respectively [4]. Other values for saponin skinned human cardiac fibers given as $[Ca^{2+}]_{50}$ are 1.06 ± 0.09 μM aequivalent to a pCa of 5.97 and $1.53 \pm 0{,}32$μM aequivalent to a pCa of 5.82 [94,99]. Reported values from triton-X 100 chemically skinned human cardiac fibers are a pCa of 5.5 and 5.67 for atrial fibers and ventricular fibers, respectively [27]. In general, slow muscles like cardiac and smooth muscle exhibit Ca^{2+}-sensitivies, which are 0.2-0.3 pCa units higher than those from fast muscles. In addition, the Ca^{2+}-sensitivity in human cardiac fibers as reported by Morano et al. [27] is 0.17 units higher in ventricular than in atrial fibers. Here, the characteristic differences seem to be mainly due to the atrial myosin containing α-MHC as opposed to the ventricular myosin which in man contains predominantly β-MHC [69].

In addition, differences in species play an important role as well experimental conditions and possible inaccuracies have a large effect on the results. The last point has been critically addressed by some authors. Comparisons in absolute numbers of data between different authors thus are critically to be considered. In the beginning of skinned fiber research, it was assumed only free Ca^{2+} would determine muscle contraction.

Table 1 gives an overview on physiological, pathophysiological and pharmacological mechanisms which all have influence on calcium sensitivity of cardiac muscle.

Increase – sensitizing effect:	
sarcomere length	[32, 38, 39]
- Phosphorylation of regulatory myosin light chain	[20]
- Carnosine	[95]
- Caffeine	[100
- Cardiotonic drugs (calcium sensitizers)	

Sulmazole (AR-L115 BS)	[16, 101]
Pimobendan (UDCG-115-BS)	[102, 103]
BM 14.478	[104]
Isomazole	[105]
EMD-53998	[106]
EMD-57033	[107]
CGP-48506	[108]
Decrease – desensitizing effect:	
Temperature	[31, 109, 110]
- Inorganic phosphate	[111, 112]
- MgATP	[113]
- Mg	[50, 113]
- Ionic strength	[114]
Phosphorylation of troponin I	[115, 43, 116, 117]
Intracellular pH/Hypoxia: Acidosis	[55, 52, 118]
shown to be regulated by TnI Hypoxia causes rapid hydrolysis of myoplasmic creatine phosphate and the accumulation of inorganic phosphate and creatine	[119]

Table 1: Sensitizing and desensitizing influences [4,11]

Figures 9 and 10 show original data of own experiments with calcium-sensitizer EMD 57033 and proteinkinase A, respectively.

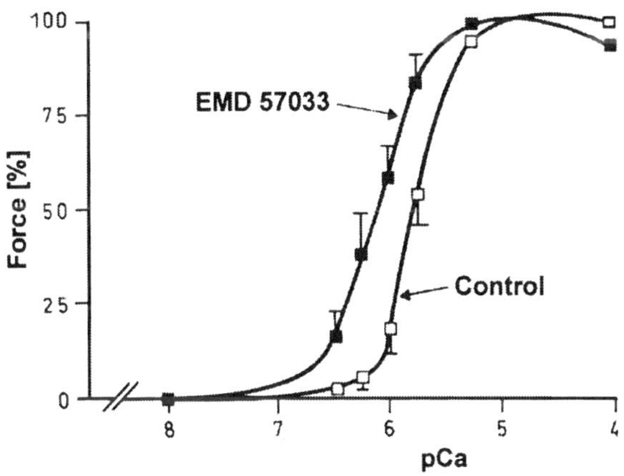

Figure 9: Influence of EMD 57033, a calcium-sensitizer on force-pCa relationship. A leftward shift of the activation curve indicates the increase in sensitivity to calcium (unpublished own experiments).

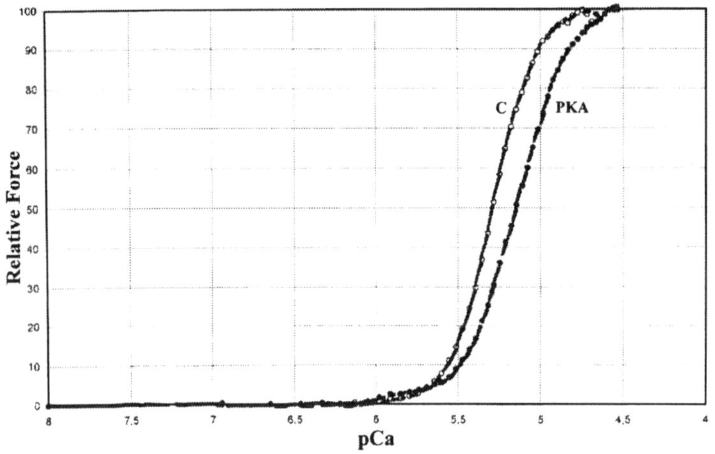

Figure 10: Force-pCa relationship in human myocardium: 3µM PKA shifts the relationship to the right, i.e., phosphorylation of contractile proteins decreases sensitivity of the contractile proteins to calcium (unpublished own experiments).

The steepness of the curve is aequivalent to the cooperativity of binding cross-bridges. *H*, the Hill coeffecient reflects this cooperativity in the pCa-tension relation. When we look at mammalian cardiac and skeletal muscle, the steepness in cardiac muscle is much lower moving in a range between 1.9 and 2.5 dependent on the specimen [4]. Skeletal muscle reaches values of 4-6. In human atrial and ventricular cardiac muscle values of 2.0 - 3.0 are reported. This reflects the fine adjustment and force regulation by changes in the Ca^{2+}-concentration (see below). Since cardiac TnC contains only one functional Ca^{2+} binding regulatory site, any value of $H > 1$ indicates cooperativity involving multiple complexes of the regulatory system on the actin filament. For activation levels up to around 20% of maximal tension, increasing Ca^{2+} seems to increase the total number of recruited cross-bridges. At higher levels of activation, Ca^{2+} seems to increase tension by affecting the cross-bridge turnover kinetics directly [91]. All reported *H* values strongly depend on physiological factors such as sarcomere length and experimental conditions [38].

5.3.3. The Sarcoplasmic Reticulum

The sarcoplasmatic reticulum (SR) seems to have reached a more important role in hearts of warm-blooded animals and in man than in fish and frog heart, in which intracellular Ca^{2+} is almost entirely controlled by the myocyte's membrane.

The SR takes part in the excitation-contraction coupling which begins with membrane depolarization. When thus voltage-sensitive Ca^{2+}-channels in the sarcolemma are activated and small amounts of Ca^{2+} enter the myocyte, Ca^{2+} release channels are activated in the adjacent junctional sarcoplasmic reticulum [119]: the resulting efflux of stored SR Ca^{2+} increases $[Ca^{2+}]_i$ and initiates contraction. The amount of Ca^{2+} released by the SR depends on the size and duration of the initial Ca^{2+} trigger. This allows $[Ca^{2+}]_i$ transient amplitudes to be graded [120] – an important feature in cardiac muscle, where all cells contract with each beat. Modulation of the $[Ca^{2+}]_i$ transient amplitude provides one mechanism to vary the force of contraction, by which cardiac output is matched to the body's metabolic demands.

It should be emphasized, here, that Fabiato and Fabiato have given the greatest approach in this field of research on SR with the skinned fiber method during the late 70ies and 80ies. As mentioned before, the SR release is triggered by induced Ca^{2+} inward currents through membrane depolarization observed in mechanically skinned cardiac myocytes [119]. But the amount of increasing $[Ca^{2+}]_i$ is not suffient to activate muscle contraction processes, directly [4]. Regarding Ca^{2+}-release from SR, Caffeine and IP_3 had an enhancing effect in skinned fiber experiments working on two different mechanisms [120], while Mg^{2+} and ruthenium inhibited caffeine induced Ca^{2+}-release [121]. A fall of pH over the range 7.4 - 6.5 directly inhibits the SR Ca^{2+}-release channel [122].Other functional different receptors in Ca^{2+}-release is the inositol-1,4,5-triphosphate receptor (IP_3R) and a third subtype of ryanodine receptor (RyR_3) [123].

After contraction, the Ca^{2+} pump immediatly removes Ca^{2+} from the cytosol into the non-junctional part of the SR mainly near the transverse tubules, at the Z-line of the sarcomere [124]. Ca^{2+}-reuptake can be influenced by pH, ATP and Mg^{2+} as skinned fiber experiments indicated [52,125]. Decreasing pH in saponin skinned rat ventricular fibers correlated with a decrease of the Ca^{2+}-reuptake by the SR. An additional effect is that Ca^{2+}-sensitivity decreases (see above). An increase in intracellular Pi independent from the mechanism of pH reduces sarcoplasmic reticular calcium loading and thus depresses the Ca^{2+}-induced Ca^{2+}-release [122]. This could be an important contributing factor in the hypoxic or ischaemic contractile failure of the myocardium. However the detrimental effect of P_i may be offset to some extent by a stimulatory action of

ADP on the calcium release mechanism of the Ca^{2+}-induced Ca^{2+}-release [126]. A slower relaxation rate could be explained on the basis of this possible mechanism. The Ca^{2+}-reuptake can be stimulated by cAMP dependent protein kinase phophorylation of phospholamban [127,128]. Dephosphorylated phopholamban is an inhibitor of the SR-Ca^{2+}-ATPase activity [128]. The impact of a decrease in SR-Ca^{2+}-ATPase activity could result in a slower relaxation. Interestingly, Rogers et al. [129] reported about PKC to decrease SERCA2 function.

But what about SR function do we want to know under physiological conditions? (i) The velocitiy and quantity of Ca^{2+}-transport, and (ii) the capacitiy of Ca^{2+} storing in the SR. To Assess the SR Ca^{2+} content, besides electron probe microanalysis, rapid cooling experiments, cumulative extracellular Ca^{2+} depletions, and direct chemical and radiotracer techniques and also the skinned fiber method were used in caffeine-induced contractures [4]. Thus Ca^{2+}-capacity estimations (μmol Ca/kg wet weight) can received by a determination with the fluorescent Ca^{2+} indicator, indo-1: values vary from larger than 57 up to ~300 reported [119,130,131,132,133].

5.3.4. Length-Tension Relation

Regarding the length-tension relationship of cardiac muscle we refer to Chapter I: The Frank-Starling mechanism.

5.3.5. ATPase Activity-Force Relation

The acto-myosin adenosine triphosphatase is the place of transformation of chemical energy stored in adenosine-triphosphate (ATP) to mechanical energy and work of the heart. It is activated at sufficient free intracellular Ca^{2+} concentrations and regulated through various mechanisms located in the contractile apparatus. In the chemical process ATP is hydrolysed to adenosine-diphosphate (ADP) and free inorganic phosphate (P_i).

In general, ATP is mainly used by the myofilaments (tension generation and cell shortening), for intracellular calcium handling, and for maintaining the intracellular milieu through ATP dependent ion transports. Important to consider in heart disease is the question for myofilament ATP consumption efficiency: For what are „costs of contraction“ payed? In heart failure, increased cardiac contractility is neccessary for pump function.

5.3.5.1 Tension-cost in mammalian myocardium

In mammalian myocardium the composition of α- and ß-myosin heavy chains may alter with age, thyroid gland activity, neurohumoral status and the load imposed on the cardiac muscle. These molecular changes are thought to change myocardial economy, i.e., the tension-cost relationship. Figure 11 demonstrates that tension-cost relation depends indeed on this composition.

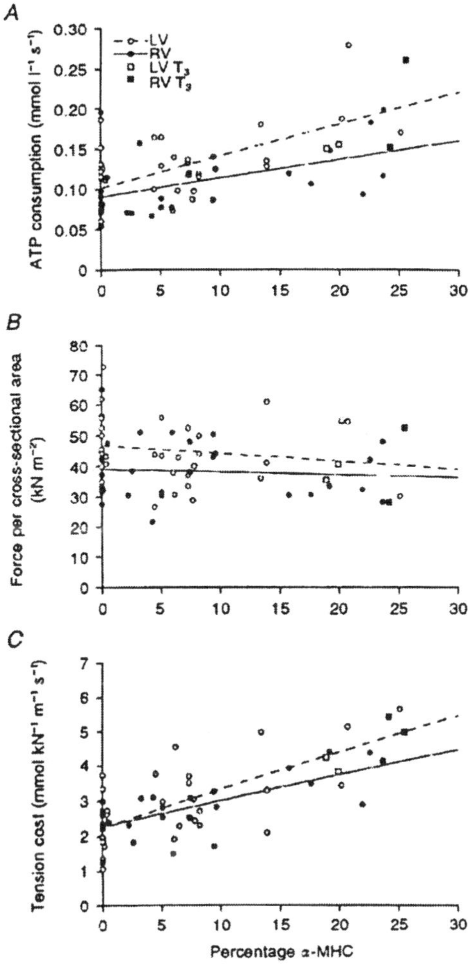

*Figure 11: ATP consumption (**A**), force development (**B**), and tension cost (**C**). Tension cost is clearly dependent on a-myosin heavy chain content. Samples were taken from the left ventricle (LV) and right ventricle (RV). In order to obtain cardiac muscle with high content of a-myosin heavy chain, guinea pigs were treated by injection of triiodo-tyronine (T_3) for one week. According to [134].*

In this study [134] the amount of α-myosin heavy chain was modulated by age and chronic application of triiodothyronine. The authors concluded that from the analysis of the linear relationship between tension-cost and percentage α-myosin heavy chain that the "slow" ß-myosin heavy chain is about five times more economical than the "fast" α-myosin heavy chain. There cannot be any doubt that changes in the α- and ß-myosin heavy chains which are neither age-dependent nor thyroid gland related but rather reflect pathophysiological states like hypertrophy and failure result in the same changes of myocardial economy as analyzed by the tension-cost relation.

Regarding ß-adrenoceptor stimulation and thereby phosphorylation of contractile proteins, the data available in the literature are conflicting: whereas Saeki and coworkers [135] were able to find a decreased economy due to application of PKA (Figure 12), de Tombe and Stienen [19] reported unchanged economy under conditions of PKA application, although both scientific groups used rat skinned cardiac fibers (see below).

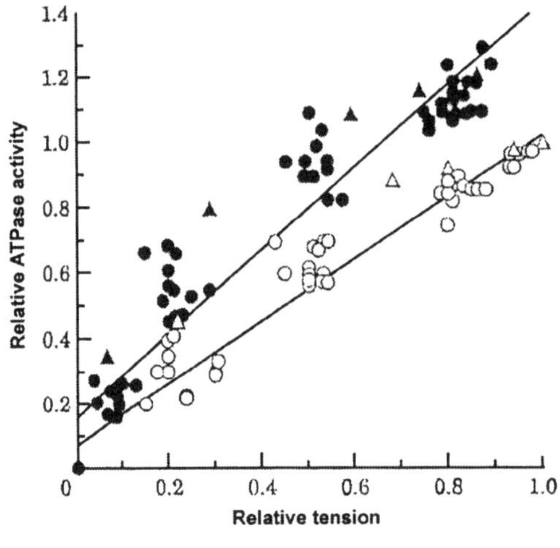

Figure 12: ATPase activity as a function of force development in skinned rat cardiac muscle. Note the increase in this ratio after exposition to PKA (filled symbols). According to [135].

5.3.5.2. Tension-cost relation in human myocardium

Regarding tension-cost relations in human myocardium, to our knowledge, only one original publication is available: In 1991, Morano et al [136] compared human atrial myocardium to human ventricular myocardium and found the ATPase versus force ratio to be at least twice as high in atrial as compared to ventricular myocardium and to be independent on pCa (Figure 13).

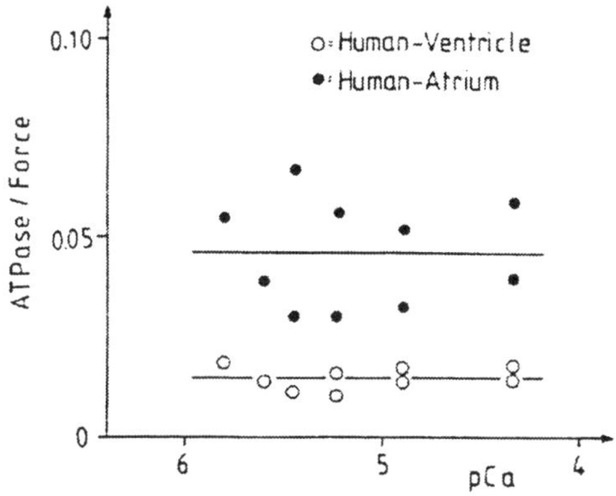

Figure 13: ATPase activity as a function of developed force in human skinned atrial and ventricular preparations. This ratio is at least twofold higher in atrial than in ventricular myocardium. According to [136].

This difference in tension-cost relationship was attributed to the clear difference in the content of α-myosin heavy chain existing between atrial and ventricular human myocardium.

Regarding acute interventions with PKA, we performed a number of experiments in human failing left ventricular myocardium. In about half of the experiments, an upward shift in the tension-cost relationship was observed (Figure 14, typical example).

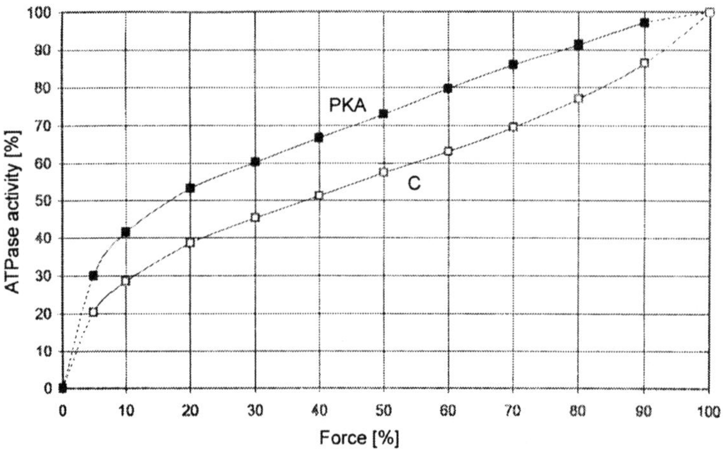

Figure 14: ATPase activity as a function of developed tension in a skinned human fibre of a failing left ventricle. In this example, PKA increases this ratio and thereby decreases economy. PKA, protein kinase A; C, control. (Own unpublished data).

However, in the other half of experiments, no change in myocardial economy could be detected. These differences in results may be related to different phosphorylation states of the diseased myocardium. Pretreatment conditions before heart transplantation (catecholamines, ß-blockers) may also play an important role.

Currently, data available compairing tension-cost relations between human failing and nonfailing myocardium are rare. Brixius et al [137] reported preliminary data stating a decreased ratio between ATPase and developed tension (Figure 15).

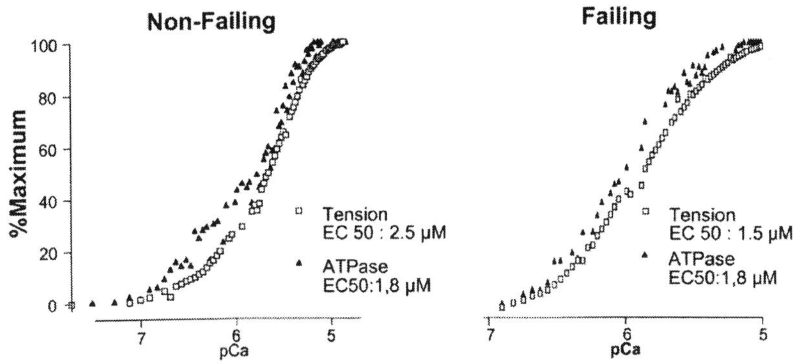

Figure 15: Tension-cost in human ventricular nonfailing ***(left)*** *and failing* ***(right)*** *myocardium. Tension is more economically generated in failing than in nonfailing human myocardium. This Figure was kindly provided by Brixius and Schwinger [137].*

5.3.5.3. Tension-cost relations with calcium sensitizers

We measured ATPase activity in human ventricular skinned fibers at different calcium concentrations before and after application of 10 µM CGP 48506. This calcium sensitizer (see Table 1 of this chapter) significantly decreased the tension-cost relation (see Figure 16) and thereby crossbridge cycling rate.

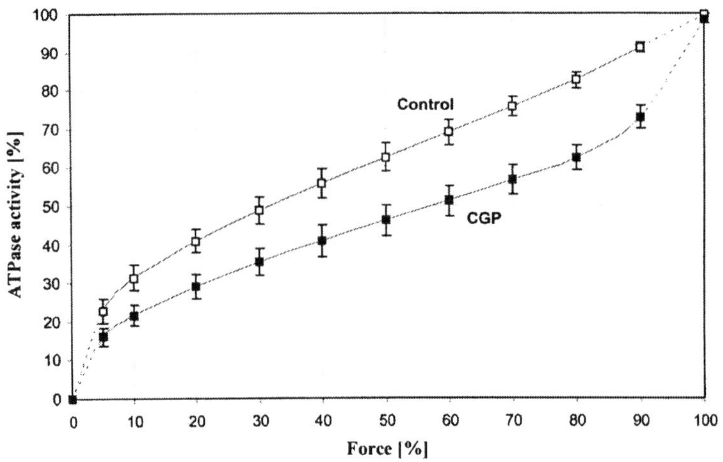

Figure 16: Tension-cost relationship before (control) and after application of 10μM CGP-48506. This calcium-sensitizer significantly shifts the relationship to the right thereby increasing economy of force generation. ATPase activity at 50% of force development is 65.5±3.7% for control and only 46.2±3.9% for CGP-48506 (n=9; p<0.005). Unpublished results.

5.4. Discussion

5.4.1. Methodological Considerations

Concerning the relation of free Ca^{2+}-concentration to actively developed force of a single muscle the named method is a gold standard in physiological muscle experiments. When showing the principle of the method, it is clear that its ultimate advantage is based on the direct impact on the contractile apparatus through used solutions. For this purpose, the cell's membranes have to be taken apart, chemically or mechanically. Since these functional multicellular preparations are a compromise between intact muscular preparations and singular contractile proteins and are examined under almost physiological conditions, there are difficulties to consider for accurate interpretation of the obtained results.

1 For inhibition of cell contracture and muscle damage during dissection the myocardium is often treated with BDM before its preparation [138]. Thus, the phosphorylation status of the myofilament proteins may be affected. That is important to consider for the interpretation of experiments on intracellular signaling [139].

2 With the skinning of muscular tissue, substances important for the contractile apparatus can get lost. These are natural sensitizers as taurin and carnosine derivates as well as partly contractile proteins themselves [89,45].

3 Unphysiologically high Ca^{2+}-solutions seem to activate proteases that destroy troponin [89].

4 In the laboratory prepared solutions can differ from the physiological intracellular liquid [32].

5 Mistakes in calculating and preparation of the used solutions have a great impact on Ca^{2+}-responsiveness. Even little alterations of the free Ca^{2+}-concentration lead to a shift in the pCa-tension relationship and false interpretations of the absolute tension development in the range of lower Ca^{2+}-concentrations [29,140,4,141].

6 Whereas the use of baths may advance fast solution changes, the gradient method provides a better opportunity to picture the whole process of activation. In the latter, little steps allow to view little changes in muscle activation.

7 The attachment of a muscle fiber to the force transducer damages the fixed ends. These may allow internal shortening of some populations of muscle cells. Aluminium clips, glue, nylon snares or metal tweezers are described for fixation [61,62,142,143].

8 The lack of the sarcolemma allows the contractile proteins to change their interfilament lattice spacings [144,110,145,58].

9 Tension development of skinned fibers from diseased hearts might be influenced by the alteration of the extracellular matrix, i.e., fibrosis occurs as a pathophysiological consequence in the failing heart [7]. Inhomogeneity of multicellular preparations complicate the interpretation of received results [146].

5.4.2. Special Considerations of ATPase Activity Measurement by Photometer Detection of NADH

The measurement of ATPase activity is possible through indirect and direct means with the skinned fiber method. Here, especially problems of direct measurement by NADH fluorescence detection are discussed, since the authors have worked with this means.

In general, adding substances as azide prevent a high ATPase signal at rest of the fiber [81] with an effect also dependent on the skinning period. There is a negligible resting activity in the presence of azide. This shows that the acto-myosin ATPase is well regulated [45]. This is in contrast with results from suspensions of isolated cardiac myofibrils obtained by homogenization, which commonly show a Ca^{2+}-independent (basal) ATPase activity that is about 10-20% of the total activity [147,148]. A resting activity of less than 30% of the total activity is acceptable. NADH loses its luminescent effect due to so-called photo-bleaching [149,19,135]. As NADH-concentration decreases, the very sensible parameter ATPase activity is more limited to detect. Therefore, after preparation the solution should be kept in a darkened, cooling box. Contamination of the LDH with NADH is discussed as another reason[135]. Stress of the fiber before the experiment has direct impact on the signal during rest [45]. This makes it more difficult to detect a clear difference of extinction at activation. It is discussed of whether there is an influence of the signal by a washing out of main regulator proteins as TnC as a main problem of skinning. Another problem is the diffusion of enzymes, NADH and Ca^{2+} in the elucidated area. The field of detection is influenced by the muscle structure, the field's size and the illumination. The smaller the field is chosen, the more stabile the signal behaves. But the area should cover the whole diameter of the cuvette [60].

Once the experiment has started, the signal is influenced by all parameters that have an impact on the Ca^{2+}-sensitivity, as we found mainly temperature. As a special problem of the gradient mixture, a differing pH of the relaxing and activating solution affects the NADH fluorescence signal with every step of influx trigger during the activation. Since there is a slow diffusion in the afferent part of the tube to the cuvette, the netto effect appears also very slow. All together, every differing parameter influencing the base line of the ATPase signal moves the background signal of non-specific ATPases below or above which has a direct impact on the extinction. However, it is also to consider that artifacts in the ATPase-force relationships may result from Pi-accumulation which is as well important for measurements of sarcomere length [150]. The time resolution of the described ATPase determination is probably limited by the time needed to exchange the solution in the cuvette and by the accurancy of the fluorescence determination rather than by the turnover frequency of the enzymatic reaction. Furthermore, a decrease of the fluorescence may be seen as a result of the washing out of contractile proteins by the solution changes [45].

Human myocardium has its own character. In this approach, there exists a difference in the intensity of the background signal in comparison to mammalian myocardium. The reason might be seen in a greater amount of non-specific ATPases or a different phosphorylation status especially possible in the failing heart [152].

5.4.3. Tension-cost and composition of α- and ß-myosin heavy chains

Studies in mammalian and human myocardium have clearly demonstrated that the distribution of the "fast" α-myosin heavy chain and "slow" ß-myosin heavy chain has clear impact on myocardial economy of contraction and thereby on crossbridge cycling mechanics. This finding is in good agreement with studies using other methods to study mechanics and energetics of the myocardium like shortening velocity (Chapter 3), myothermal approach (Chapter 4), and the frequency-response method (Chapter 6). The lack of α–myosin heavy chain gene expression in the failing human myocardium [153,154] clearly indicates a decreased ATPase versus tension ratio, i.e., improved economy of myocardial contraction in the diseased heart (own preliminary data and [137]). One might argue that the content of α-myosin heavy chains in human left ventricular nonfailing myocardium is quite small [153,154], and therefore, might not play a role in contraction kinetics and economy. However, one has to realize that the "fast" α-myosin heavy chain has a fivefold higher tension-cost relation than the "slow" ß-myosin heavy chain. Therefore, even a small percentage of α-myosin heavy chain (see Figure 11 according to [134]) might significantly alter the tension-cost relation.

For many years, a decreased tension-cost relation has been considered to be beneficial from an energy saving point of view. However, as outlined in the discussion of Chapters 4 and 6, slower and more economical muscles have decreased power output which may contribute to failure of heart muscle. Therefore, it might be wise to search for pharmacological tools which act via stimulation of gene expression of α-myosin heavy chains, for example, the carnitin-palmitoyl-transferase inhibitor etomoxir [155].

5.4.4. Tension-cost and PKA stimulation

Regarding the tension-cost consequences of phosphorylation of contractile proteins by PKA, the results are very conflicting. Because the skinned fiber preparation is very delicate regarding washout of substances, and alterations of the phosphorylation status may result from disease, pretreatment of patients prior to heart transplatation, and from specific handling of the preparation itself, we do belief that phosporylation has significant influence on the tension-cost ratio. This view is based on (1) our own experience (see Figure 14 in this Chapter) and (2) on the fact that other methodological approaches do show alteration of crossbridge kinetics due to phosphorylation (see Chapter 4, the myothermal approach, and Chapter VI, the frequency-response method).

REFERENCES

1) Lymn RW, Taylor LR: Mechansism of adenosine triphosphate hydrolysis by actomyosin. Biochemistry 1971:10; 4617-4624

2) Ford LE, Huxley AF, Simmons MR: Tension responses to sudden length change stimulated frog muscle fibres near slack length. J Physiol (Lond) 1977;269:441-515

3) Brenner B: The cross-bridge cycle in muscle. Mechanical, biochemical and structural studies on single rabbit psoas fibers to characterize cross.bridge kinetics in muscle for correlation with the actomyosin-ATPase in solution. Basic Res Cardiol 1986: 1-15

4) Bers DM: Excitation-Contraction Coupling and Cardiac Contractile Force. (ed) Dordrecht / Boston / London 1991: Kluwer Academic Publishers

6) Holubarsch C, Lüdemann J, Wiesner S, Ruf T, Schulte-Baukloh H, Schmidt-Schweda S, Pieske B, Posival H, Just H: Shortening versus isometric contractions in isolated human failing and non-failing left ventricular myocardium: dependency of external work and force on muscle length, heart rate and inotropic stimulation. Cardiovasc Res 1998;37(1): 46-57

7) De Tombe PP: Altered contractile function in heart failure. Cardiovasc Res 1998;37(2): 367-80

8) Parmley, WW: Pathophysiology of Congestive Heart Failure. Am J Cardiol 1985;56:7A-11A

9) Holubarsch Ch, G. Hasenfuss, H. Just, E. M. Blanchard, L. A. Mulieri, N. R. Alpert: Modulation of myothermal economy of isometric force generation by positive inotropic interventions in the guinea pig myocardium. Cardioscience 1990;1:33-41

10) Holubarsch, C: New inotropic concepts: rationale for and differences between calcium sensitizers and phosphodiesterase inhibitors. Cardiology 1997;88(Suppl 2):12-20

11) Rüegg JC ed: Calcium in muscle activation. In:Calcium in Muscle Activation. Berlin Heidelberg New York 1986: Springer pp.6-28, 43-45, 59-81, 165-200

12) Bers DM: Excitation-Contraction Coupling and Cardiac Contractile Force. (ed) Dordrecht / Boston / London 1991: Kluwer Academic Publishers

13) Solaro RJ, Pang DC, Briggs FN: The purification of cardiac myofibrils with Triton X-100. Biochim Biophys Acta 1971;245:259-62

14) Rüegg JC, Morano I: Calcium-sensitivity modulation of cardiac myofibrillar proteins. J Cardiovasc Pharmacol 1989;14(Suppl 3):S20-3

15) Saida K, Nonomura Y: Characteristics of Ca2+ an Mg2+ induced tension development in chemically skinned smooth fibers. J Gen Physiol 1978;72:1-14

16) Herzig JW, Feile K, Rüegg RC: Activating effects of AR-L 115 BS on the Ca^{2+} sensitive force, stiffness and unloaded shortening velocity (Vmax) in isolated contractile structures from mammalian heart muscle. Arzneim Forsch/Drug Res 1981; 31: 188-191

17) Fawcett JM, Harrison SM, Orchard CH: A method for reversible permeabilization of isolated rat ventricular myocytes. Exp Physiol 19981; 83:293-303

19) De Tombe PP, Stienen GJ: Protein kinase A does not alter economy of force maintenance in skinned rat cardiac trabeculae. Circ Res 1995;76:734-41

20) Morano I, Hofmann F, Zimmer M, Rüegg JC: The influence of P-light chain phosphorylation by myosin light chain kinase on the calcium sensitivity of chemically skinned heart fibres. FEBS Lett 1985; 189:221-4

21) Nayler W, Merrillees N: Some observations on the fine structure and metabolic activity of normal and glycerinated ventricular muscle of toad. J Cell Biol 1964;22:533-550

22) Fabiato A, Fabiato F: Activation of skinned cardiac cells. Subcellular effects of cardioactive drugs. Eur J Cardiol 1973;1:143-55

23) Stienen GJ, Güth K, Rüegg JC: Force and force transients in skeletal muscle fibres of the frog skinned by freeze-drying. Pflugers Arch 1983; 397:272-6

24) Podolsky RJ: Membrane systems in muscle cells. In: Aspects of cell motility. Symposia of the Society for Experimental Biology. University Press, Cambridge 1968:87-99

25) Blanchard EM, Pan BS, Solaro RJ: The effect of acidic pH on the ATPase activity and troponin Ca^{2+} binding of rabbit skeletal myofilaments. J Biol Chem 1984;259:3181-6

26) Leijendekker WJ, Herzig JW: Reduction of cross-bridge turnover rate in the presence of EMD 52998, a novel Ca^{2+}-sensitizing agent. Pflugers Arch 1992;421:388-390

27) Morano I, Arndt H, Gartner C, Rüegg JC: Skinned fibers of human atrium and ventricle: myosin isoenzymes and contractility. Circ Res 1988;62:632-9

28) Kitada Y, Narimatsu A: Increase in Ca^{2+}-sensitivity of contractile system by MCI-154, a novel cardiotonic agent, in chemically skinned fibres from the guinea pig papillary muscles. J Pharmacol Exp Ther 1987;243:633-638

29) Miller DJ, Smith GL: EGTA purity and the buffering of calcium ions in physiological solutions. Am J Physiol 1984;246:C160-C166

30) Fabiato A, Fabiato F: Calculator programs for computing the composition of the solutions containing multiple metals and ligands used for experiments in skinned muscle cells. J Physiol 1979;75:463-505

31) Godt RE, Lindley BD: Influence of temperature upon contractile activation and isometric force production in mechanically skinned muscle fibers of the frog. J Gen Physiol 1982;80:279-97

32) Hibberd MG, Jewell BR: Calcium- and length-dependent force production in rat ventricular muscle. J Physiol (Lond) 1982;329:527-40

33) Bers DM: A simple method for the accurate determination of free [Ca^{2+}] in Ca-EGTA solutions. Am J Physiol 1982;242:C404-C408

34) Harrison SM, Bers DM: Correction of absolute stability constants of EGTA for temperature and ionic strength. Am J Physiol 1989;258:C274-C281

35) Brandt PW, Cox RN, Kawai M, Robinson T: Effect of cross-bridge kinetics on apparent Ca^{2+} sensitivity. J Gen Physiol 1982;79: 997-1016

36) Lee JA, Allen DG (eds): Modulation of cardiac calcium sensitivity. A new approach to increasing the strength of the heart. Oxford University Press 1993

37) Thames MD, Teichholz LE, Podolsky RJ: Ionic strength and the contraction kinetics of skinned muscle fibers. J Gen Physiol 1974;63: 509-30

38) Kentish JC, Ter Keurs HEDJ, Ricciardi L, Bucx JJJ, Noble MIM: Comparison between the sarcomere length-force relations of intact and skinned trabecuae from rat right ventricle. Circ Res 1986;58:755-768

39) Allen DG, Kentish JC: The cellular basis of the length-tension relation in cardiac muscle.J Mol Cell Cardiol 1985;17:821-840

40) Solaro RJ, Briggs FN: Estimating the functional capabilities of sarcoplasic reticulum in cardiac muscle. Circ Res 1974;34:531-540

41) Endo M, Kitazawa T: E-C coupling on skinned cardiac fibres. In: Biophysical aspects of cardiac muscle. M Morad, ed. Academic Press, New York 1977:307-327

42) McClellan GB, Winegrad S: The regulation of the calcium sensitivity of the contractile system in mammalian cardiac muscle. J Gen Physiol 1978;72:737-64

43) Hellam DC, Podolsky RJ: Force measurements in skinned muscle fibres. J Physiol 1969;200:807-819

44) Kentish JC, Stienen GJM: Differential effects of length on maximum force production and myofibrillar ATPase activity in rat skinned cardiac muscle. J Physiol (Lond) 1994;475:175-84

45) Kerrick WG, Donaldson SKB: The comparative effects of [Ca2+] and [Mg2+] on tension generation in the fibers of skinned frog skeletal muscle and mechanically disrupted rat ventricular cardiac muscle. Pflugers Arch 1975; 358:195-201

46) Ventura-Clapier R, Mekhfi H, Vassort G:). Role of creatine kinase in force development in chemically skinned rat cardiac muscle. J Gen Physiol 1987;89:815-37

47a) Natori R: The property and contraction process of isolated myofibrils. Jikeikai Med J 1954;1:119-126

47b) Grimm AF, Whitehorn WV: Characteristics of resting tension of myocardium and localization of its elements. Am J Physiol 1966;210:1362-1368

48) Fabiato A: Calcium release in skinned cardiac cells: variations with species, tissues, and development. Fed Proc 1982;41: 2238-44

49) Fabiato A, Fabiato F: Dependence of the contractile activation of skinned cardiac cells on the sarcomere length. Nature 1975;256:54-6

50) Fabiato A, Fabiato F: Effects of magnesium on contractile activation of skinned cardiac cells. J Physiol (Lond) 1975;249:497-517

51) Fabiato A, Fabiato F: Dependence of calcium release, tension generation and restoring forces on sarcomere length in skinned cardiac cells. Eur J Cardiol 1976;4 (Suppl):13-27

52) Fabiato A, Fabiato F: Effects of pH on the myofilaments and the sarcoplasmic reticulum of skinned cells from cardiace and skeletal muscles. J Physiol (Lond) 1978;276: 233-55

53) Szent-Györgyi A: Free energy relations and contraction of actomyosin. Bio Bull (Woods Hole) 1949;96:140-161

54) Weber HH, Portzehl H: The transference of the muscle energy in the contraction cycle. Prog Biophys Mol Biol 1954;4:60-111

55) Schädler M: Proportionale Aktivierung von ATPase-Aktivität und Kontraktionsspannung durch Calciumionen in isolierten kontraktilen Strukturen verschiedener Muskelarten. Pflügers Arch 1967;296:70-90

56) Portzehl H, Caldwell PC, Rüegg JC: The dependence of contraction and relaxation of muscle fibers from crab Maia squinado on the internal concentration of free calcium ions. Biochim Biophys Acta 1964;79:581-591

57) Arndt H, Katus HA, Mall G, Rüegg JC: Different calcium sensitivity and mechanical properties of skinned fibres from hypertrophic and non-hypertrophic atria. Muscle Res Cell Motil 1987;8:75

58) Watkins H, Seidman CE, Seidman JC, Feng HS, Sweeney HL: Expression and functional assessment of a truncated cardiac troponin T that causes hypertrophic cardiomyopathy. Evidence for a dominant negative action. J Clin Invest 1996;98:2456-2461

58) Godt RE, Maughan DW: Swelling of skinned muscle fibers of the frog. Experimental observations. Biophys J 1977;19:103-16

59) Ford LE, Huxley AF, Simmons RM: Tension response to sudden length change in stimulated frog muscle fibres near slack length. J Physiol 1977;269:441-515

60) Güth K, Wojciechowski R: Perfusion cuvette for the simultaneous measurement of mechanical, optical and energetic parameters of skinned muscle fibres. Pflugers Arch 1986;407: 552-7

61) Goldman YE, Simmons RM: Control of sarcomere length in skinned muscle fibres of rana temporaria during mechanical transients. J Physiol 1984;350:497-518

62) Wolff MR, Whitsell LF, Moss RL: Calcium Sensitivity of Isometric Tension Is Increased in Canine Experimetnal Heart Failure. Circ Res 1995;76:781-789

63) Palmer S, Kentish JC: Roles of Ca2+ and crossbridge kinetics in determining the maximum rates of Ca2+ activation and relaxation in rat and guinea pig skinned trabeculae. Circ Res 1998;83:179-86

64) Ashley CC, Moicescu DG, Rose RM: Aequorin-light and tension responses from bundles of myofibrils following a sudden change in free calcium. J Physiol 1974;241:104P-196P

65) Moisescu DG: Kinetics of reaction in calcium-activated skinned muscle fibres. Nature 1976;262:610-3

66) Blinks JR, Wier WG, Hess P: Measurement of Ca2+ concentrations in living cells. Prog Biophys Mol Biol 1982;40:1-114

68) Fawcett DW, McNutt NS: The ultrastructure of the cat myocardium I. Ventricular papillary muscle. J Cell Biol 1969;42:1-45

69) Schaub MC, Hefti MA, Zuellig RA, Morano I: Modulation of contractility in human cardiac hypertrophy by myosin essential light chain isoforms. Cardiovasc Res 1998;37:381-404

70) Huxley AF: Low-angle diffraction studies on muscle. Disc Faraday Soc 1951;11:148

71) Brenner B: Sarcomeric domain organization within single skinned rabbit psoas fibers and its effects on laser light diffraction patterns. Biophys J 1985;48:967-82

72) Goodship-Patience R, Hibbert MG, Jewell BR: Apparatus for studying the mechanical properties of skinned muscle fibres. Proc Physiol Soc 1979;290:P13-P14

73) Gordon AM, Pollack GH: Effects of calcium on the sarcomere length-tension relation in rat cardiac muscle. Circ Res 1980;47:610-619

74) Fenn WO: A quantitiative comparison between the energy liberated and the work performed by the isolated sartorius muscle of the frog. J Physiol 1923;58:175-203

75) Fenn WO: The relation between the work performed and the energy liberated in muscular contraction. J Physiol 1924;58:373-395

76) Hill AV: Myothermic experiment on a frog gastrocnemius. Proc Roy Soc London Ser B 1931;107:115-131

77) Hill AV: Heat of shortening and the dynamic constants of muscle. Proc Royal Soc 1938;126:136

78) Edman KAP: The velocity of unloaded shortening and its relation to sarcomere length and isometric force in vertebrate muscle fibers. J Physiol (Lond) 1979;291:143-159

79) Goldman YE, Hibberd MG, McGray JA, Trentham DR: Relaxation of muscle fibres by photolysis of caged ATP. Nature 1982;300:701-5

80) Huxley AF: Muscle Structure and theories of contraction. Prog Biophys 1957;144:403-425

81) Stienen GJ, Roosemalen MC, Wilson MG, Elzinga G: Depression of force by phosphate in skinned skeletal muscle fibers of the frog. Am J Physiol 1990;259:C349-57

82) Zot HG, Güth K, Potter JD: Measurement of fluorescence and tension development in skinned skeletal muscle fibers reconstituted with TnCDanz. Biophys J 1985;47:473

83) Güth K, Winnikes K, Potter JD: Cycling cross-bridges increase the Ca2+ affinity to TnC. Biophys J 1986;49:270a

84) Dantzig JA, Goldman YE, Millar NC, Lacktis J, Homsher E: Reversal of the cross-bridge force-generating trasition by photogeneration of phophate in rabbit psoas muscle fibres. J Physiol 1992;451:247-278

85) Brenner B, Yu LC: Structural changes in the actomyosin cross-bridges associated with force generation. Proc Natl Acad Sci USA 1993;90:5252-6

86) Brenner B: Effect of Ca2+ on cross-bridge turnover kinetics in skinned single rabbit psoas fibers: implications for regulation of muscle contraction. Proc Natl Acad Sci USA 1988;85:3265-9

87) Moss RL: Ca2+-regulation of mechanical properties of striated muscle: mechanistic studies using extraction and replacement of regulatory proteins. Circ Res 1992;70:865-884

87) Siemankowski RF, White HD: ADP dissociation from actomyosin subfragment 1 is sufficiently slow to limit the unloaded shortening velocity in vertebrate muscle. Proc Natl Acad Sci USA 1985;82:658-662

88) Barry WH, Bridge JHB: Intracellular calcium homeostasis in cardiac myocytes. Circulation 1993;87:1806-1815

89) Gao W, Backx PH, Azan-Backx M, Marban E: Myofilament sensitivity in intact versus skinned rat ventricular muscle. Circ Res 1994;74:408-415

90) Hill AV: The possible effects of the aggregation of the molecules and haemoglobin on its dissociation curves. Nature 1910;90:4-7

91) Tobacman LS: Thin filament-mediated regulation of cardiac contraction. Annu Rev Physiol 1996;58:447-481

92) Wier WG, Yue DT: The effect of 1,4-dihydropyridine type Ca2+-channel antagnists and agonists on intracellular [Ca2+] transients accompanying twitch contraction of heart muscle. In: Fleckenstein A, Breemen C van, Groß R, Hoffmeister F (eds) Cardiovascular effects of dihydropyridine-type calcium antagonists and agonists. Springer, Berlin Heidelberg New York 1985:188-197

94) Hajjar RJ, Gwathmey JK: Cross-bridge dynamics in human ventricular myocardium. Regulation of contractility in the failing heart [published erratum appears in Circulation 1994 Jan;89(1):509]. Circulation 1992;86:1819-26

95) Harrison SM, Lamont C, Miller DJ: Carnosine and other natural imidazoles enhance muscle Ca-sensitivity and are mimicked by caffeine and AR-L 115BS. J Physiol 1986;371:197P

96) Fabiato A: Myoplasmic free calcium concentration reached during the twitch of an intact isolated cardiac cell and during calcium-induced release of calcium from sarcoplasmic reticulum of a skinned cardiac cell from adult rat or rabbit ventricle. J Gen Physiol 1981;78:457-497

97) Hofmann PA, Fuchs F: Effect of length and cross-bridge attachment on Ca2+ binding to cardiac troponin C. Am J Physiol 1987;253:C90-6

98) Hofmann PA, Fuchs F: Evidence for a force-dependent component of calcium binding to cardiac troponin C. Am J Physiol 1987;253:C541-6

99) Hajjar RJ, Grossman W, Gwathmey JK: Responsiveness of the myofilaments to Ca2+ in human heart failure: implications for Ca2+ and force regulation. Basic Res Cardiol 1992;87(Suppl 1):143-59

100) Wendt IR, Stephenson DG: Effects of caffeine on Ca-activated force production in skinned cardiac and skeletal muscle fibres of the rat. Pflügers Arch 1983;398:210-216

101) Solaro RJ, Rüegg JC: Stimulation of Ca2+ binding and ATPase activity of dog cardiac myofibrils by AR-L 115 BS, a novel cardiotonic agent. Circ Res 1982;51:290-294

102) Rüegg JC, Pfitzer G, Eubler D, Zeugner C: Effect on contractility of skinned fibres from mammalian heart and smooth muscle by a new benzimidazole derivative, [4,5-dihydro-6-2-(4-methoxyphenyl)-1H-benzimidazol-5-yl]-5-methyl-3(2H)-pyridazinone. Arzneim Forsch / Drug Res 1984;34:1736-1738

103) Fujino K, Sperlakis N, Solaro RJ: Sensitization of dog and guinea pig heart myofilaments to Ca2+ activation and the inotropic effect of pimobendan: Comparison with milrinone. Circ Res 1988;63:911-922

104) Müller-Beckmann B, Sponer G, Rüegg JC, Freund P, Jäger H, Strein K: Zur Pharmakologie der neuen positiv inotropen Substanzen BM 14.478. Z Kardiol 1986;75 (Suppl IV):31

105) Lues I, Siegel R, Harding J: Effect of isomazole on the responsiveness to calcium of the contractile elements in skinned cardiac muscle fibres of various species. Eur J Pharmacol 1988;146:145-153

106) Beier N, Harting J: The novel cardiotonic agent EMD 53998 is a potent 'calcium sensitizer'. J Cardiovasc Pharmac 1991;18:17-27

108) Herold P, Herzig JW, Wenk P, Leutert T, Zbinden P, Fuhrer W, Stutz S, Schenker K, Meier M, Rihs M: 5-Methyl-6-phenyl-1,3,5,6-tetrahydro-3,6-methano-1,5-benza-diazocine-2,4-dione (BA 41899): representative of a novel class purely calcium-sensitizing agents. J Med Chem 1995;38:2946

109) Harrison SM, Bers DM: Influence of temperature on the calcium sensitivity of the myofilaments of skinned ventricular muscle from the rabbit. J Gen Physiol 1989;93:411-28

110) Harrison SM, Bers DM: Modification of temperature dependence of myofilament Ca sensitivity by troponin C replacement. Am J Physiol 1990;258:C282-8

111) Herzig JW, Ruegg JC: Myocardial cross-bridge activity and its regulation by Ca++, phosphate and stretch. In: Riecker G, et al., ed. Myocardial failure. Berlin, Springer 1977: 41-51

112) Kentish JC: The effects of inorganic phosphate and creatine phosphate on force production in skinned muscles from rat ventricle. J Physiol (Lond) 1986;370:585-604

113) Best PM, Donaldson SKB, Kerrick WGL: Tension in mechanically disrupted mammalian cardiac cells: Effects of magnesium adenosine triphosphate. J Physiol 1977;265:1-17

114) Kentish JC: The inhibitory effects of monovalent ions on force development in detergent-skinned ventricular muscle from guinea-pig. J Physiol (Lond) 1984;352:353-74

115) Mope L, McClellan GB, Winegrad S: Calcium sensitivity of the contractile system and phosphorylation of troponin in hyperpermeable cardiac cells. J Gen Physiol 1980;75:271-282

116) Holroyde MJ, Howe E, Solaro RJ: Modification of calcium requirements for activation of cardiac myofibrillar ATPase by cyclic AMP dependent phosphorylation. Biochim Biophys Acta 1979;586:63-69

117) Herzig JW, Kohler G, Pfitzer G, Rüegg JC, Wölffle G: Cyclic AMP inhibits contractility of detergent treated glycerol extracted cardiac muscle. Pflugers Arch 1981;391:208-12

118) Blanchard EM, Solaro RJ: Inhibition of the activation and troponin calcium binding of dog cardiac myofibrils by acidic pH. Circ Res 1984;55:382-91

119) Fabiato A: Calcium-induced release of calcium from the cardiac sarcoplasmic reticulum. Am J Physiol 1983;245:C1-14

119) Wattanapermpool J, Reiser PJ, Solaro RJ: Troponin I isoforms and differential effects of acidic pH on soleus and cardiac myofilaments. Am J Physiol 1995;268:C323-30

120) Fabiato A: Two kinds of calcium-induced release of calcium from the sarcoplasmic reticulum of skinned cardiac cells. Adv Exp Med Biol 1992;311:245-62

120) Stern MD, Lakatta EK: Excitation-contraction coupling in the heart: the state of the question. Faseb J 1992;6:3092-100

121) Rousseau E, Meissner G: Single cardiac sarcoplasmic reticulum Ca2+-release channel: Activation by caffeine. Am J Physiol 1989:256:H328-H333

122) Kentish JC, Xiang JZ: Ca(2+)- and caffeine-induced Ca2+ release from the sarcoplasmic reticulum in rat skinned trabeculae: effects of pH and Pi. Cardiovasc Res 1997;33:314-23

123) Marks AR: Intracellular Calcium release channels: regulators of life and death. Am J Physiol 1997;272:597-605

124) Jorgensen AO, Shen AC-Y, Daly P, MacLennan DH: Localization of Ca2+ and Mg2+-ATPase of the sarcoplasmatic reticulum in adult rat papillary muscle. J Cell Biol 1982;93:883-892

125) Fabiato A: Simulated calcium current can both cause calcium loading in and trigger calcium release from the sarcoplasmic reticulum of a skinned canine cardiac Purkinje cell. J Gen Physiol 1985;85:291-320

126) Xiang JZ, Kentish JC: Effects of inorganic phosphate and ADP on calcium handling by the sarcoplasmic reticulum in rat skinned cardiac muscles. Cardiovasc Res 1995;29:391-400

127) Sasaki T, Inui M, Kimura Y, Kuzuya T, Tada M: Molecular mechanisms of regulation of Ca2+ pump ATPase by phospholamban in cardiac sarcoplasmic reticulum: effects of synthetic phospholamban peptides on Ca2+ pump ATPase. J Biol Chem 1992;267:1674-1679

128) James P, Inui M, Tada M, Chiesi M, Carofoli E: Nature and site of phospholamban regulation of the Ca2+ pump of sarcoplasmic reticulum. Nature 1989;342:90-92

129) Rogers TB, Gaa ST, Massey C, Dosemeci D: Protein kinase C inhibits Ca2+ accumulation in cardiac sarcoplasmic reticulum. J Biol Chem 1990;265:4302-4308

130) Hunter DR, Haworth RA, Berkoffet HA: Measurement of rapidly exchangeable cellular calcium in the perfused beating rat heart. Proc Nat Acad Sci USA 1981;78:5665-5668

131) Bers DM: SR Ca loading in cardiac muscle preparations based on rapid cooling contractures. Am J Physiol 1989;256:C109-C120

132) Solaro RJ, Briggs FN: Estimating the functional capabilities of sarcoplasic reticulum in cardiac muscle. Circ Res 1974;34:531-540

133) Dani AM, Cittadini A, Inesi G: Calcium transport and contractile activity in dissociated mammalian heart cells. Am J Physiol 1979;237:C147-C155

134) Van der Velden J, Moorman AF, Stienen GJM: Age-dependent changes in myosin composition correlate with enhanced economy of contraction in guinea-pig hearts. J Physiol (Lond) 1998;507:497-510

135) Saeki Y, Kobayashi T, Minamisawa S, Sugi H: Protein kinase A increases the tension cost and unloaded shortening velocity in skinned rat cardiac muscle. J Mol Cell Cardiol 1997;29:1655-63

136) Morano I, Bletz C, Wojciechowsky R, Rüegg JC: Modulation of crossbridge kinetics by myosin isoenzymes in skinned human heart fibers. Circ Res 1991;68:614-8

137) Brixius K, Sarridou-Zaroh P, Reuter H, Schwinger RHG: Impaired length dependent tension development and myosin-ATPase activity in failing human myocardium. Circulation 1999 (Suppl I);100:305

138) Pate E, Cooke R: Addition of phosphate to active muscle fibers probes actomyosin states within the powerstroke. Pflugers Arch 1989;414:73-81

139) Venema RC, Kuo JF: Protein kinase C-mediated phosphorylation of troponin I and C-protein in isolated myocardial cells is associated with inhibition of myofibrillar actomyosin MgATPase. J Biol Chem 1993;268:2705-2711

140) Solaro RJ, Lee AE, Kentish JC, Allen DG: Effects of acidosis on ventricular muscle from adult and neonatal rats. Circ Res 1988;63:779-787

141) Seow CY, Ford LE: High ionic strength and low pH detain activated skinned rabbit skeletal muscle cross-bridges in low force state. J Gen Physiol 1993;101:487-511

142) Palmer S, Kentish JC: Differential effects of the Ca2+ sensitizers caffeine and CGP 48506 on the relaxation rate of rat skinned cardiac trabeculae. Circ Res 1997;80:682-7

143) Krueger JW, Pollack GH: Myocardial sarcomere dynamics during isometric contraction. J Physiol 1975;251:627-643

144) Jewell BR: A reexamination of the influence of muscle length on myocardial performance. Circ Res 1977;40:221-30

145) De Beer EL, Grundeman RLF, Wilhelm AJ, van den Berg C, Caljouw CJ, Klepper D, Schiereck P: Effect of sarcomere length and filament lattice spacing on force development in skinned cardiac and skeletal muscle preparations from the rabbit. Bas Res Cardiol 1988;83:410-423

146) McDonald M, Wolff R, Moss RL: Force-velocity and power-load curves in rat skinned cardiac myocytes. J Physiol 1998;511:519-531

147) Solaro RJ, Shiner JS: Modulation of Ca2+ control of dog and rabbit cardiac myofibrils by Mg2+. Comparison with rabbit skeletal myofibrils. Circ Res 1976;39:8-14

148) Kentish JC, Nayler WG: The influence of pH on the Ca2+-regulated ATPase of cardiac and white skeletal myofibrils. J Mol Cell Cardiol 1979;11:611-7

149) Stienen GJ, Papp Z, Elzinga G: Calcium modulates the influence of length changes on the myofibrillar adenosine triphosphatase activity in rat skinned cardiac trabeculae. Pflugers Arch 1993;425:199-207

150) Kawai M, Güth K, Winnikes K, Haist C, Rüegg JC: The effect of inorganic phosphate on the ATP hydrolysis rate and the tension transients in chemically skinned rabbit psoas fibers. Pflugers Arch 1987;4081-9

151) Griffiths PJ, Güth K, Kuhn HJ, Rüegg JC: ATPase activity in rapidly activated skinned muscle fibres. Pflugers Arch 1980;387:167-73

152) Wolff MR, Buck SH, et al.: Myofibrillar calcium sensitivity of isometric tension is increased in human dilated cardiomyopathies: role of altered beta-adrenergically mediated protein phosphorylation. J Clin Invest 1996;98:167-76

153) Lowes BD, Minobe W, Abraham WT, et al.: Changes in gene expression in the intact human heart. Downregulation of a-myosin heavy chain in hypertrophied, failing ventricular myocardium. J Clin Invest 1997;100:2315-2324

154) Nakao K, Minobe W, Roden R, Bristow WR, Leinwand LA: Myosin heavy chain gene expression in human heart failure. J Clin Invest 1997;2370-2372

155) Schmidt-Schweda S, Holubarsch Ch: First clinical trial with etomoxir in patients with chronic congestive heart failure. Clinical Science 2000;99:27-35

6. THE FREQUENCY RESPONSE METHOD

6.1. Introduction

The intrinsic speed of myocardial shortening, an important biological variable, is known to be different between species and chambers and to be subject of alteration due to metabolic/hormonal status and hemodynamic conditions. Usually, speed of contraction is measured during twitches of cardiac muscle opposed to different afterloads. However, the results from isotonic shortening experiments depend not only on the properties of the contractile proteins but also – to a great part – on the excitation-contraction coupling [1,2]. Especially, the time-dependence of the active state of the muscle may have fundamental influence on the measured velocities.

Therefore, as a more direct approach to changes in the intrinsic speed of cardiac contractile proteins more specific methods are necessary which are independent on the processes involving excitation-contraction coupling.

The frequency method can be used as a unique means which can be applied to any given system in order to study its dynamic properties. This method has been applied to skeletal and – later on – cardiac muscle by changing the muscle length sinusoidally with a fixed small amplitude using a variety of frequencies. Plotting the amplitude ratio and phase relation of force response waves to length change waves as a function of frequency yields a fundamental description of the dynamic properties of a muscle which is called *transfer function analysis*.

6.2. Methods

The frequency response method may be used either in skinned fiber preparations [3] or in non-skinned myocardial preparations in barium contracture [4]. Both approaches have in common the steady state of the activation of contractile proteins: Constant calcium concentration in skinned fibers and permanent activation by barium ions. Using barium contracture, one might argue that this procedure might influence cardiac dynamics in an unexpected way on the one hand; using skinning solutions, on the other hand, this procedure might also have some impact on the interaction between actin and myosin. In an elegant study performed by Saeki et al., compatibility was demonstrated for results obtained from non-skinned (barium contracture) and chemically skinned (calcium activation) preparations [5].

To successfully perform transfer function analysis, some requirements of the apparatus are necessary. The longitudinal muscle preparation must be attached to a force transducer with high resonance frequency (~6 kHz) and a linear motor which is driven by a sinus function generator (for example Muscle Research System, Scientific Instruments, Heidelberg, Germany). Length changes of the muscle can be derived from the linear motor.

Figure 1 demonstrates the effect of calcium withdrawal and barium application.

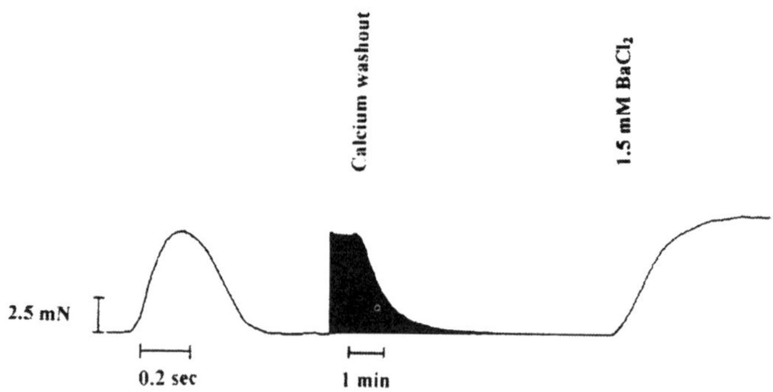

Figure 1: Human muscle strip Preparation: ***Left:*** *Single twitch due to electrical stimulation.* ***Middle:*** *Reduction of force amplitude due to calcium washout.* ***Right:*** *Application of bariumchloride induces stable barium contracture.*

Figure 2 shows typical experiment of a cardiac muscle under study (barium contracture) and Figure 3 the respective data analysis.

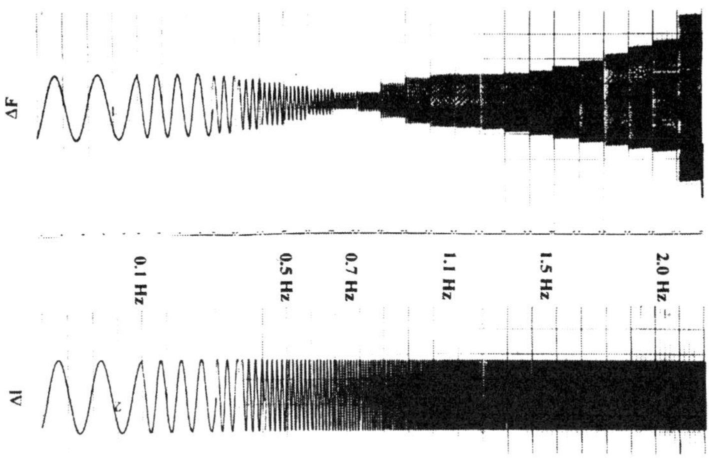

Figure 2: The frequency-response experiment in a left ventricular muscle strip preparation. Note the constant sinusoidal change in length Δl, but a dip in the change in force ΔF at 0.7 Hz.

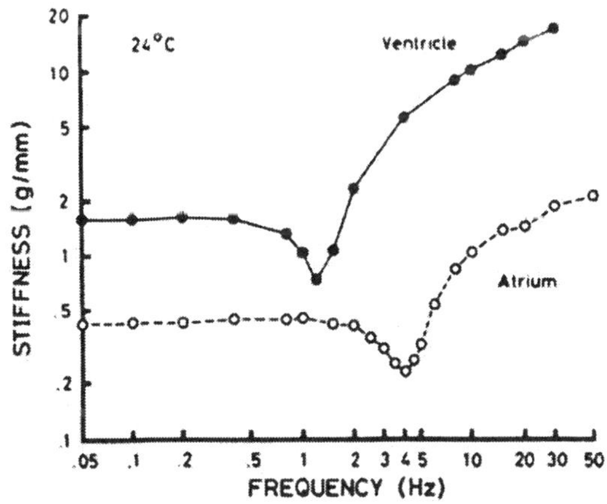

Figure 3: Stiffness, $\Delta F/\Delta l$, plotted as a function of frequency. Note that minimum stiffness frequency is different between atrial and ventricular myocardium. According to [10].

In contrast to previous reports [6,7], in which the minimum stiffness frequency (f_{min}) was thought to be determined solely by the crossbridge cycling rate, Berman et al. [8] discussed and Campbell et al. [9] mathematically analyzed the phenomenon of the minimum stiffness frequency as the interaction between crossbridge recruitment dynamics and crossbridge cycling dynamics: At low oscillating frequencies, the ratio between force-generating and non-force-generating crossbridges is stabile. Therefore, the changes in force are proportional to the changes in length due to recruitment of a greater number of crossbridges, according to the Frank-Starling mechanism. When the oscillating frequency increases, there is a critical frequency at which the time for complete recruitment will be too short within a single oscillation. As a consequence, stiffness must decrease because of the reduced ratio between force-generating and non-force-generating crossbridges. At higher oscillating frequencies, beyond the dip (minimum frequency f_{min}), cycling crossbridges are significantly distorted by rapid length changes before regular crossbridge detachment can occur.

The best way to test the sensitivity and reliability of the frequency response method is to alter fundamental biophysical parameters which are believed to have either maximum effect on crossbridge dynamics, i.e., experimental temperature, or zero effect on crossbridge dynamics, i.e., cardiac muscle length according to the Frank-Starling mechanism (see Chapter I). There is general agreement that minimum frequency is temperature-dependent by a Q_{10}-factor of around 3 (Figure 4) [10,11,12] demonstrating the biochemical energy-dependent basis for the behavior of minimum stiffness frequency.

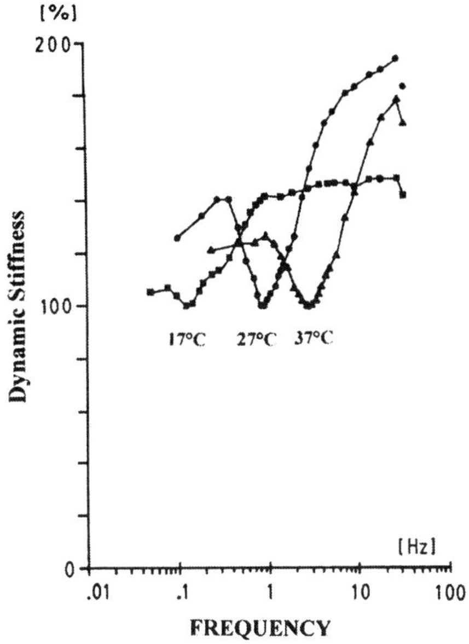

Figure 4: Left ventricular muscle strip preparation at 17°, 27°, and 37°C. Dip frequency changes with experimental temperature (Q_{10} ~ 2.7). According to [12].

Changes in muscle length which are thought to have influence on the number of force-generating crossbridges (degree of overlap; calcium sensitivity) but not on the dynamics of a single crossbridge had no effect on minimum stiffness frequency (see Figure 5) [10].

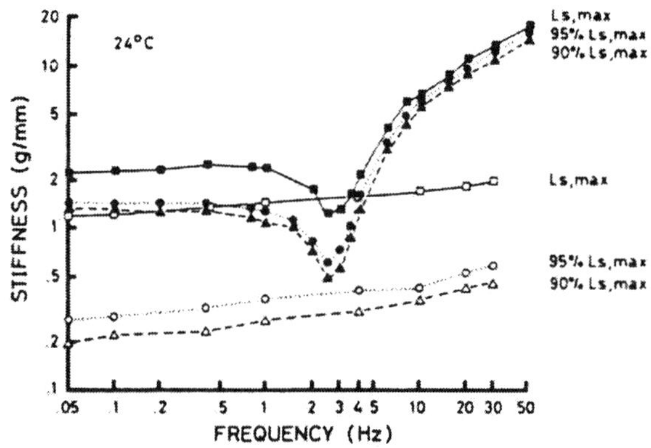

Figure 5: Length of the muscle has no influence on dip frequency. Solid symbols show curves for barium contracture at three different muscle lengths; open symbols represent data obtained from the same muscle at rest. According to [10].

6.3. Results

The results section is subdivided into four parts: A. Experiments with animal myocardium. Acute interventions. B. Experiments with animal myocardium. Chronic changes. C. Experiments with human myocardium. Acute interventions. D. Experiments with human myocardium. Chronic changes.

6.3.1. Experiments with Animal Myocardium. Acute Interventions

The effect of β_1-adrenoceptor stimulation on minimum stiffness frequency has been studied in rabbit [8] and in rat papillary muscle [13]. Both authors used preparations in barium contracture. However, whereas Berman et al. [8] applied sinusoidal length changes, Hoh et al. [13] applied pseudo-random binary noise-modulated perturbations. Nevertheless, the results were quite similar: β_1-adrenoceptor stimulation exhibited a 23 % increase in minimum frequency in rabbit myocardium and a 49 % increase in minimum frequency in normal rat myocardium (Figure 6 [13]).

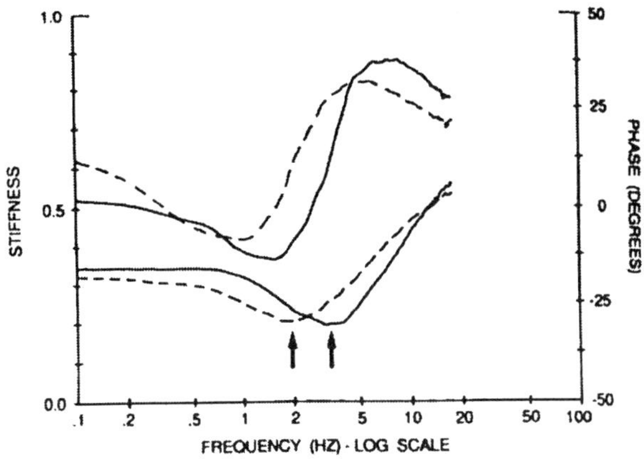

Figure 6: Dynamic stiffness as a function of frequency and phase plots obtained from normal rat myocardium (V_1) before and after (—) application of 0.3μM adrenaline. According to [13].

Interestingly, when rats were made hypothyrotic by treatment with propylthiouracil, and, thereby, the myosin isoenzymes were shifted to almost pure V3, the effect of adrenaline on increase of minimum frequency was only 26 % as compared to 49 % in euthyrotic rats with almost pure V1 myocardium [13]. In another study, Hoh et al., demonstrated that dibutyryl cyclic AMP and xanthine derivatives both of which increase intracellular cyclic AMP, had the same increasing effect on minimum frequency as adrenaline. In contrast, ouabain did not alter the stiffness spectrum [14].

6.3.2. Experiments with Animal Myocardium. Chronic Changes

There are two reports in the literature investigating dynamic stiffness of animal myocardium using the length-perturbation method: Rossmanith et al. [15] report a minimum frequency of 2.1 Hz in V1 containing rat myocardium (normal) and of 1.1 Hz in V3 containing rat myocardium (hypothyrotic). Shibata et al. [10] measured values for mininum frequency of 0.8 Hz in normal rabbit myocardium (V3) and of 2.5 Hz in thyrotoxic rabbit myocardium (V1). These authors were also able to demonstrate fundamental differences in minimum frequency between adult and newborn, and between ventricular and atrial myocardium [10]. A summary of their data is given in Figure 7 [10].

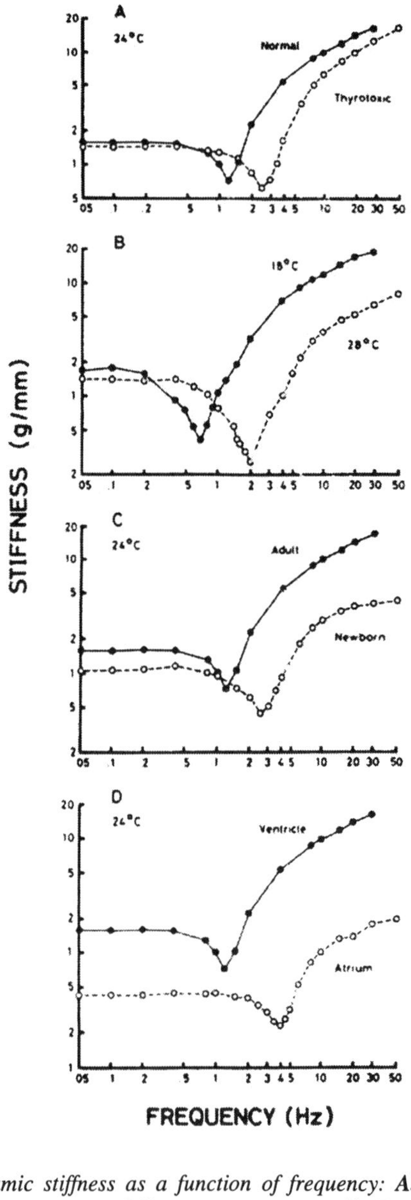

Figure 7: Dynamic stiffness as a function of frequency: ***A.*** *Thyrotoxic versus normal cardiac muscle.* ***B.*** *Experiments at different temperatures.* ***C.*** *Experiments performed with adult and newborn myocardium.* ***D.*** *Comparison between atrial and ventricular myocardium. According to [10].*

6.3.3. Experiments with Human Myocardium. Acute Interventions

To our knowledge, there is only one study available investigating the effect of a β_1-adrenoceptor agonist on crossbridge mechanics in human myocardium using the length perturbation method. In this study, isoproterenol shifted the minimum frequency in n=16 out of n=19 individual experiments significantly to higher values. Altogether, a significant shift of +18 % was observed (see Figure 8) [12].

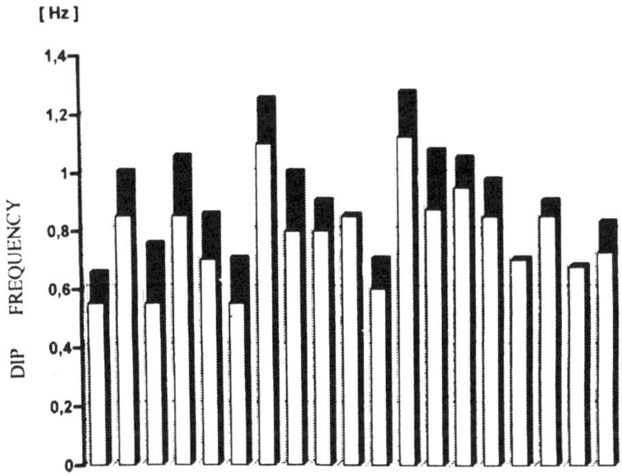

Figure 8: Increase in dip frequency due to isoproterenol application in 19 preparations obtained from human left ventricles. According to [12].

Interestingly, this shift of minimum frequency was associated with a significant decline in contracture force (for interpretation see Discussion).

6.3.4. Experiments with Human Myocardium. Chronic Changes

Using chemically skinned muscle fibers from failing and non-failing human myocardium in combination with the frequency response method, Hajjar and Gwathmay were able to demonstrate a clear difference between control (normal) and myopathic (diseased) human myocardium [17] (Figure 9).

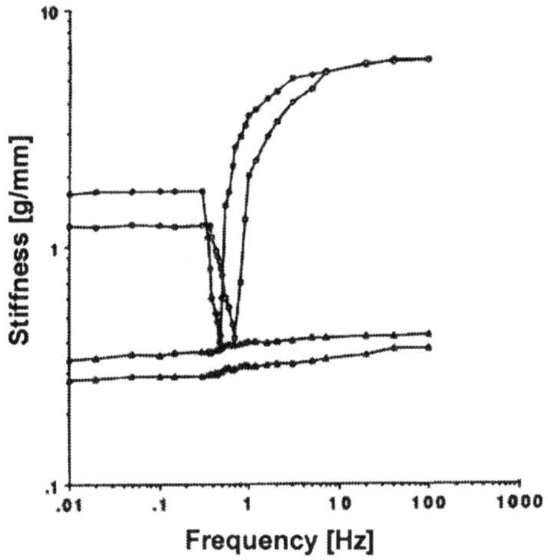

Figure 9: In human failing myocardium (solid symbols), dip frequency is shifted to lower frequencies compared to normal myocardium (open symbols). According to [16].

At 22 °C experimental temperature, minimum frequency was 0.78 Hz in normal and 0.42 Hz in myopathic muscles. These results are in good agreement with those of Ruf et al. [12] using an experimental temperature of 27 °C: These authors found a minimum frequency of 1.1 Hz in control and of 0.78 Hz in diseased human myocardium.

6.4. Discussion

Independent on species (animal or human) as well as disease (hypothyroidism or heart failure), stimulation of β_1-adrenoceptors leads to a shift of minimum frequency towards higher values. It may well be that in the diseased myocardium such an effect may attenuated due to downregulation of β_1-adrenoceptors and other alterations of the signal transduction system taking place in heart failure. This may explain the fact that three human failing myocardial preparations did not show any response to isoproterenol (Figure 8).

It is of special interest that the increase in minimum stiffness frequency is associated with a decrease in contracture force. This association of crossbridge mechanics and force development may be explained in two different ways:

(1) β_1-adrenoceptor stimulation leads to phosphorylation of TnI [17,18] and, thereby, to a desensitization of the contractile machinery for calcium and barium ions. With less barium bound to TnC, the activation of the actomyosin would fall to a sub-maximum level.

(2) The observed increase in cycling rate due to catecholamines is a consequence of an increased off-rate of crossbridges from the force-generating position. However, with increased off-rate, the steady state between force-generating and non-force-generating state of crossbridges would be shifted in favor of the non-force-generating state and thereby lessen the total number of force-generating crossbridges per unit of time.

We favor the second explanation for a number of reasons: First of all, the second hypothesis explains both observations, i.e., decrease in minimum stiffness frequency and decrease in contracture force. Secondary, the first hypothesis is unlikely, because desensitization is expected to reduce muscle force only at sub-maximum concentrations of calcium or barium; at supra-maximum concentrations, a drop in maximum contracture force is unlikely to occur due to desensitization. Third, using the myothermal method (see Chapter IV) a decrease in the force-time integral was found for animal experimental studies supporting the hypothesis of a reduction of the off-rate, g_{app}, of crossbridges due to β_1-adrenoceptor stimulation. The fact that myothermal studies conducted with failing and non-failing human myocardium [19] did not show acute changes of crossbridge kinetics is not consistent with this view and needs further clarification.

Regarding chronic changes of crossbridge kinetics in hypertophy and failure as well as some hormonal and metabolic diseases, these changes occur in animal as well as human myocardium. A detailed discussion of potential molecular mechanisms underlying these changes has been given in Chapter IV. Again, we would like to stress that these alterations may have positive aspects in the sense of better economy of force generation for slower myocardium but also detrimental aspects in the sense of decreased power output. The force-velocity relation of slow and fast muscles, and how the intrinsic velocity has impact on maximum power output is shown in Figure 21 of Chapter IV. How important the plasticity of a muscle system is for general biology is demonstrated in Figure 10: A toad needs strong but slow muscles to carry the heavy weight of body and thorax; a frog needs fast muscles for a high jump lifting a low body weight quickly.

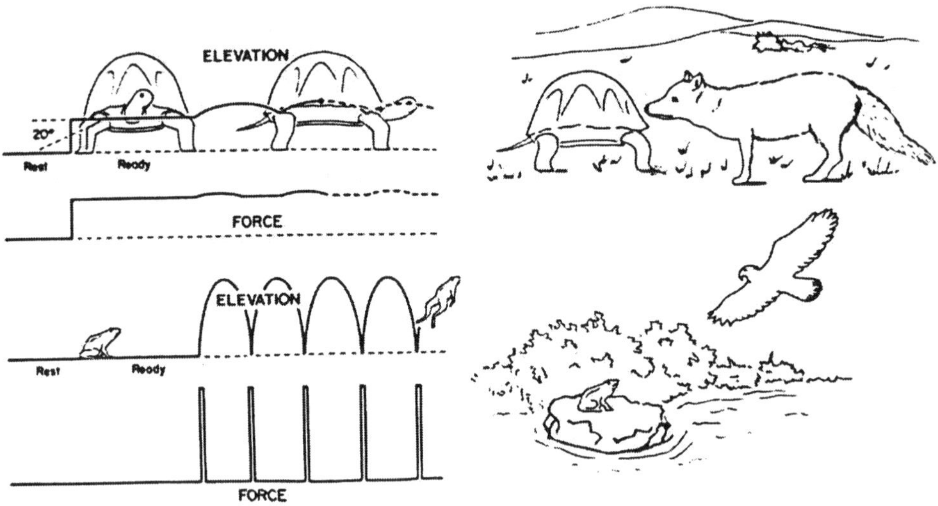

Figure 10: In general biology, there is plasticity of the muscle system: There is need for strong but slow muscles in a toad, but fast muscles in a frog. According to [20].

Compared to the broad range of plasticity of skeletal muscle (like in one species or one individual), the plasticity of heart muscle is quite small; however, changes may occur acutely (faster velocity) and chronically (slower velocity).

REFERENCES

1) Sonnenblick EH: Force-velocity relations in mammalian heart muscle. Am J Physiol 1962;202:931-939

2) Brutsaert DL, Claes VA, Sonnenblick EH: Velocity of shortening of unloaded heart muscle and the length-tension relation. Circ Res 1971;29:63-75

3) Berman MR, Lord CC, Maughan DW: Force transient time course in heart muscle with high and low V_1 to V_3 myosin isoenzyme ratio. J Moll Cell Cardiol 1988;20:679-687

4) Steiger GJ, Brady AJ, Tau ST: Intrinsic regulatory properties of contractility in the myocardium. Circ Res 1987;42:339-350

5) Saeki Y, Kawai M, Zhao Y: Comparison of crossbridge dynamics between intact and skinned myocardium from ferret right ventricles. Circ Res 1991;68:772-781

6) Kawai M, Brandt PW: Sinusoidal analysis: A high resolution method for correlating biochemical reactions with physiological process in activated muscles of rabbit, frog and cray fish. J Muscle Res Cell Motil 1980;1:279-303

7) Rossmanith H: Tension response of muscles to n-step pseudo random length reversals: A frequency domain representation. J Muscle Res Cell Motil 1986;7:299-306

8) Berman MR, Peterson JN, Yue DT, Hunter WC: Effect of isoproterenol on force transient time course and on stiffness spectra in rabbit papillary muscle in barium contracture. J Mol Cel Cardiol 1988;20:415-426

9) Campbell KB, Taheri H, Kirkpatrick RD, Burton T, Hunter WC: Simularities between dynamic elastance of left ventricular chamber and papillary muscle of rabbit heart. Am J Physiol 1993;264:H1926-H1943

10) Shibata T, Hunter WC, Sagawa K: Dynamic stiffness of barium-contracted cardiac muscles with different speeds of contraction. Circ Res 1987;60:770-779

11) Saeki Y, Sagawa K, Suga H: Dynamic stiffness of cat heart muscle in Ba^{2+}-induced contracture. Circ Res 1978;42:324-333

12) Ruf T, Schulte-Baukloh H, Lüdemann J, Posival H, Beyersdorf F, Just H, Holubarsch Ch: Alterations of crossbridge kinetics in human atrial and ventricular myocardium. Cardiovascular Res 1998;40:580-590

13) Hoh JFY, Rossmanith GH, Kwan LJ, Hamilton AM: Adrenaline increases the rat of cycling of crossbridges in rat cardiac muscle as measured by pseudo-random binary noise-modulated perturbation analysis. Circ Res 1988;62:452-461

14) Hoh JFY, Rossmanith GH, Hamilton AM: Effects of dibutyryl cyclic AMP, ouabain, and xanthine derivatives on crossbridge kinetics in rat cardiac muscle. Circ Res 1991;68:702-713

15) Rossmanith GH, Hoh IFY, Kirman A, Kwan LJ: Influence of V_1 and V_3 isomyosins on the mechanical behaviour of rat papillary muscle as studied by pseudo-random binary noise modulated length perturbations. J Muscle Res Cell Motil 1986;7:307-319

16) Hajjar RJ, Gwathmey JK: Crossbridge dynamics in human ventricular myocardium. Regulation of contractility in the failing heart. Circulation 1992;86:1819-1826

17) England PJ: Studies on the phosphorylation of the inhibitory subunit of troponin during modification of contraction in perfused rat heart. Biochem J 1976;160:295-304

18) Solaro RJ, Moir AJG, Pery SV: Phosphorylation of troponin I and the inotropic effect of adrenaline in the perfused rabbit heart. Nature 1976;262:615-617

19) Hasenfuss G, Mulieri LA, Allen PD, Just H, Alpert NR: Influence of isoproterenol and oubain on excitation-contraction coupling, crossbridge function, and energetics in failing human myocardium. Circulation 1996;94:3155-3160

20) Alpert NR, Mulieri LA, Hasenfuss G, Holubarsch Ch: Optimization of myocardial function. Basic Res Cardiol 1993;88 (Suppl 2):29-41

7. SINGLE CELL EXPERIMENTS

7.1. Introduction

Investigation on the contractile performance of non-failing and diseased myocardium was always in the center of interest in research for heart failure. For some experimental protocols it is of importance to exclude all factors, which could change the inotropic response of the examined myocardial structures. Endothelial cells and fibroblasts, which are present in large numbers in multicellular preparations like muscle strips or papillary muscles, may be responsible for these unpredictable changes of contractility. Therefore, big effort was made to develop a method, which concentrates on the contractile behaviour of one single cardiomyocyte.

Whereas papillary muscle preparations and smaller muscle strip preparations were available for a long time (see Chapter III), it was only 1981 when Powell et al. isolated intact human ventricular cardiomyocytes from children and adults for the first time [1]. They used an enzymatic approach for isolation, however, they were not able to stimulate the isolated cells. Bustamente et al. isolated atrial myocytes by a slightly changed enzymatic method and were the first to show response of human myocytes to electrical stimulation [2]. Different groups improved the method by using collagenase [3], hyaluronidase [4] and protease [5]. Cultured cardiomyocytes turned out to be very suitable for the single cell method as well.

In the meanwhile the method has been developed to a very high standard. In addition to investigations of contractile behaviour there are several sophisticated possibilities, e.g. simultaneous calcium measurements or patch clamp methods.

7.2. Methodological setup for isolated single cells

Knowing about different methodological approaches for isolating single cells as well as the measurement of single cells' contractions, this chapter is especially focused on the setup that is established in our laboratory. Isolation of cardiomyocytes differs between species. In this chapter, only isolation of human atrial and ventricular cardiomyocytes is considered.

7.2.1. Myocardial tissues and special solutions

We obtained human right atrial myocardial tissues during routine aorto-coronary bypass surgery. Left ventricular myocardial tissues could be obtained from patients, which suffered from end-stage heart failure and had to undergo heart transplantation. Non-failing myocardial tissue was restricted to hearts, which could not be transplanted for technical reasons. In addition, it is possible to isolate myocytes out of biopsies, which could be obtained during right ventricular heart catheterization.

7.2.2. Transportation of myocardial tissues

The correct storage of myocardial tissue immediately after taking the sample is a very important factor to obtain intact isolated cardiomyocytes. For this purpose we used a modified tyrode solution saturated by carbogen gas (95 % O_2 / 5 % CO_2). This solution contained (in mM) Na^+ 144, K^+ 5.8, Cl^- 126, HCO^{3-} 25, Mg^{2+} 0.96, $H_2PO_4^-$ 1.3, SO_4^{2-} 0.96, Ca^{2+} 1.25, glucose 11.2, insulin 10 U (H-Insulin, Hoechst AG) and butanedione-monoxime (BDM) 30mM. pH is adjusted to 7.4. BDM is only added during transportation and preparation of the samples. During this time the samples are especially sensitive for contractures which are caused by calcium overload provoked by cutting injuries. BDM was shown to protect the myocardium at the time of dissection [6,7].

7.2.3. Isolation of cardiomyocytes

We use the "chunk"-method for isolation of the cardiomyocytes. The tissue samples are placed in a large silicone-coated petri dish containing the carbogen saturated modified tyrode solution mentioned above. Tyrode solution should be at room temperature. It is important to remove infarcted areas and other fibrotic tissues. The samples were cut into pieces of approximately 1 mm^3 in size by means of a razor blade. This had to be done as atraumatic as possible to avoid unnecessary calcium release. Best results were obtained using a stereo-microscope for preparation.

The obtained tissue chunks are washed in a low calcium solution containing (in mM) Na^+ 120, K^+ 5,4, Cl^- 126, Mg^{2+} 5, SO_4^{2-} 5, Ca^{2+} 0,035, pyruvate 5, taurin 20, HEPES 10, glucose 0,02 at pH 7,4 for 12 min. The low calcium solution has to be saturated with carbogen gas and changed at three minutes intervals for fresh, oxygenated low calcium medium.

For enzymatic isolation three steps are necessary each lasting 45 min. Enzyme solution is prepared out of low calcium solution by adding BDM 20 mM and Ca^{2+} 0.35 mM. The pH is adjusted to 7.1. Chunks are transferred in the first step to 10 ml enzyme solution containing protease (SIGMA; ventricular tissue 3.07 U/ml, atrial tissue 4.3 U/ml). The supernatant is discarded and the chunks are resuspended in 10 ml of enzyme solution containing collagenase (Boehringer; ventricular tissue 0,21 U/ml, atrial tissue 0,27 U/ml). This second step is repeated twice. At the first incubation with collagenase, hyaluronidase (Sigma; 160 U/ml) is added only in case of isolation of atrial myocytes. This step is not necessary with ventricular tissues because of the different structure of the tissues. After 45 min the solution is put on ice for stopping enzyme activity. Isolated cells could be found in the supernatant. The portion of morphologically intact cells was between 10 and 30, rarely 50 percent.

Occasionally, myocardial tissues are not dissolved satisfactoryly after the second incubation with collagenase and only a few isolated cells can be found in the supernatant. In these cases, a third or even fourth incubation step with collagenase brings sometimes better results.

Beside this „classical" way of isolating myocytes, it is possible to gain myocytes by perfusing a part of the left ventricular wall with enzyme solution through the artery branch. This method is more expensive, but the yield of cells is normally much higher.

7.2.4. Technical setup

The technical setup for measuring the contractility of isolated single cardiomyocytes was constructed by Prof. K. Güth, Scientific Instruments, Heidelberg. In summary, it may be said that cells can be detected by a camera connected with an inverted microscope. By means of a personal computer, each single contraction can be measured and evaluated (Figure 1).

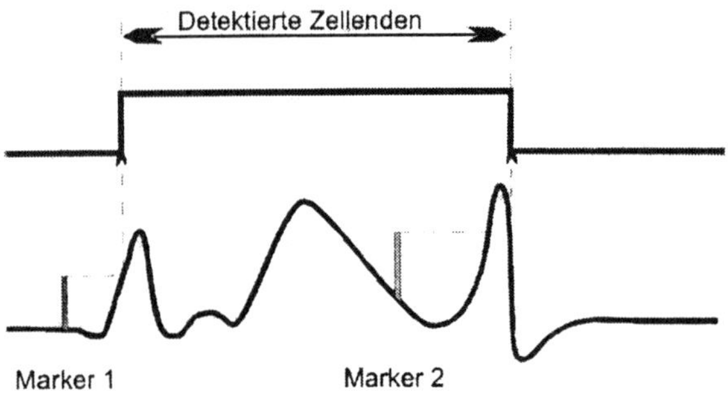

Figure 1: Detection of cell ends by use of two markers allows measurement of cell length by converting light signals to analog signals on the oszilloscop.

Microscope and cuvette system

We use an inverted phase contrast microscope (Nikon Diaphot 300). A cuvette system (Figure 2) is part of the microscope.

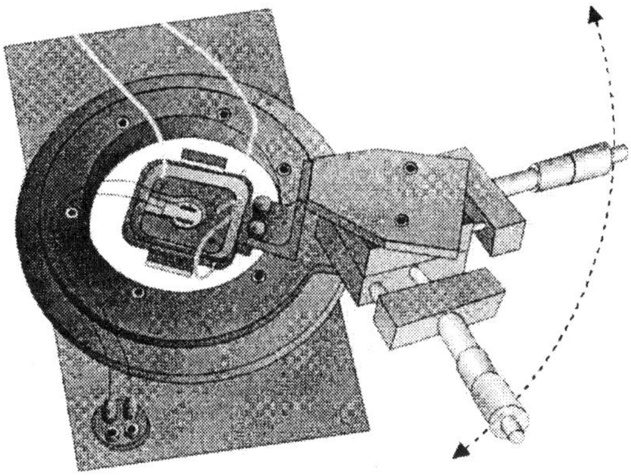

Figure 2: The organ bath integrated into a rotating cuvette table.

A probe of the supernatant with isolated myocytes is poured into the cuvette. By means of an included mirror system isolated myocytes are visible in the microscope on the one hand, and can be detected by the camera on the other hand.

The cuvette is perfused with tyrode solution using an adjustable pump. If experiments are performed at other than room temperature, the entire cuvette system had to be heated to the same temperature like the tyrode solution. In order to achieve that the temperature at the location of the cell is as close as possible to the adjusted temperature and to avoid condensation, the temperature of the objective underneath the cuvette is also feedback controlled.

Detection of cell edges

The correct detection of the cell length is indispensable in order to get trustworthy experiments. By using a phase contrast objective, the edges of the cell are well characterized by distinct transitions in brightness in reference to the background. The distances of these transitions are measured by a diode array, which is connected to the camera unit. The cell is to be brought into a line with the diode array. Therefore the cuvette system and camera unit can be rotated (Figures 2 and 3).

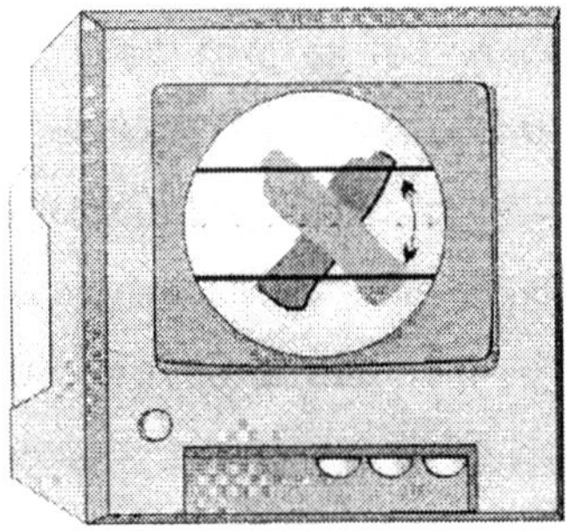

Figure 3: The rotating cuvette table allows optimal position of a single muscle cell in parallel with the diode chain.

Stimulation

Electrical stimulation of isolated cells is accomplished through platinum electrodes fitted into the cuvette system. A bipolar stimulating impulse with a duration of 5 ms is used. A voltage of 18-25 V is normally sufficient; however, some cells require voltage up to 60 V to start with contractions. In general, myocytes do not tolerate highly increasing voltage; therefore, voltage was usually adjusted only 10 % above the threshold which made cells begin to contract. To avoid gas production in terms of electrolysis at the platinum electrodes, no higher voltage and longer stimulating durations as described above should be used.

Cells do not tolerate physiological frequencies for a long period. Therefore a baseline frequency of 0.2 Hz is chosen to prevent distortion of the experiment.

Registration of contractions

The diode array detects any changes of the cell's length. By means of a connected oscilloscope and an analog-digital converter, cell length and contraction parameters could be measured and displayed on a personal computer. The software took an average of three to five single contractions in order to keep artefacts to a minimum.

The following parameters were used to evaluate the experiments:

- relative cell shortening [%]
- time to peak contraction (TTP) [ms]
- time from 10 % contraction to peak contraction ($T_{10\%}TP$) [ms]
- maximum velocity of shortening (slope max down) [-µm/s]
- maximum velocity of relaxation (slope max up) [µm/s]
- time to 50 % relaxation ($RT_{50\%}$) [ms]

General requirements

Before starting an experiment, the cuvette system is to be perfused with tyrode solution (Ca^{2+} [1.25 mM]) for at least 30 min. It turned out that this time is necessary to wash out BDM and to provide the cell with extracellular calcium ions. A cell is selected for study using the following criteria:

(1) Morphology: intact transverse striation, no vacuoles, no visible contractures
(2) No spontaneous contractions when unstimulated in 1.25 mM calcium
(3) Stable contraction amplitude and diastolic length at a stimulation rate of 0.2 Hz in 1.25 mM calcium over a period of ten minutes
(4) Only cells which contracted in line with their long axis should be used
(5) Relative cell shortening on basal conditions must exceed 2 %

If morphologically good looking cells do not react to electrical stimulation after one hour of perfusion with 1.25 mM Ca^{2+} tyrode, another attempt can be made with higher extracellular calcium concentrations. For this purpose, we stepwise increase the concentration to 1.8 mM and 2.5 mM, respectively. It is important to note that only experiments with the same tyrode's calcium concentration can be compared to each other.

If the effect of substances on the contraction behaviour of the isolated cell is tested, the substance had to be added in the tyrode reservoir. Cells are perfused and incubated for at least ten minutes, before further contractions are evaluated.

Calcium measurements

In addition to measurements of fractional shortening and contraction parameters, the single cell method is very suitable for investigations on calcium homeostasis. The intracellular calcium concentration can be estimated with calcium sensitive fluorescence indicators like indo-1 or FURA-2. These indicators are calcium chelators and change the wavelength of emitted fluorescence when binding to calcium. The fluorescent light can be collected by the objective lens and transmitted to a special spectrofluorometer for simultaneous measurement of both wavelengths. The ratio of these two wavelengths indicates the amount of bound and free calcium in the cell. Thereby, diastolic and systolic changes of intracellular calcium can elegantly be measured. The methods are described in detail elsewhere [8,9]. There are two different approaches for getting the calcium indicator into the cell: (a) Using the patch clamp method, cells can be loaded directly with the indicator salt by internal perfusion through diffusion from the micropipette. This method does not allow simultaneous contraction measurements because of sarcolemmal damage caused by the micropipette. (b) For protocols that require extracellular stimulation and contraction measurements, the cell can be loaded through the use of the membrane permeant form, an ester of the fluorescence indicator (FURA-2 AM). This ester is able to pass the sarcolemma. After loading the cell with the indicator, the cells must be washed with a tyrode solution to allow complete deesterification of the trapped dye. It must be considered that the indicators have chelating functions which lead to a loss of functional free calcium. Therefore, experiments with fluoresecence indicators should not be compared directly with experiments performed without the indicator.

It is possible to determine the exact amount of intracellular calcium by calibration of the fluorescence signals. However, it turned out that this is a very sophisticated method and it is very complicated to perform calibration with simultaneous contraction measurements.

7.3. Results

7.3.1. Influence of extracellular calcium concentration

The extracellular calcium concentration has a profound influence on the contractile behaviour of isolated cardiomyocytes. Our results (Figure 4) indicate a dose dependent increase of fractional shortening with higher extracellular calcium concentrations.

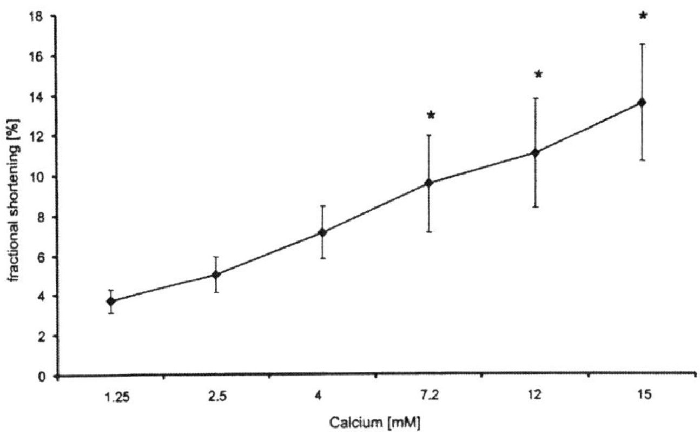

Figure 4: Fractional shortening [%] as a function of calcium concentration [mM]. 15 mM calcium increased extent of shortening by more than 200 %.

These experiments were performed using isolated left ventricular cardiomyocytes from end-stage failing human hearts. A calcium concentration of 15 mM (vs. 1.25 mM basal) led to an increase in fractional shortening by 269 %. These higher calcium concentrations also caused changes in all contraction parameters: While TTP and the velocities of shortening and relaxation were significant higher, the $RT_{50\%}$ was shown to be slightly reduced. The diastolic cell length decreased continuously with higher extracellular calcium concentrations (from 130±8 to 100±8 µm). Figure 5 shows an original registration of an isolated cardiomyocyte at $[Ca^{2+}]_o$ 1.25 mM and $[Ca^{2+}]_o$ 15 mM.

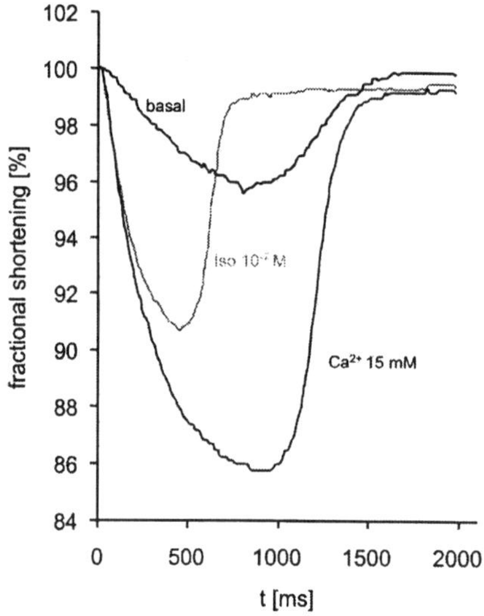

Figure 5: Original records of a myocyte under basal, isoproterenol (10^{-7} M) and high calcium (15 mM) conditions. Both isoproterenol and high calcium increase the extent of shortening; however, isoproterenol profoundly shortens time of contraction compared to basal and high calcium.

Similar results concerning fractional shortening were obtained by Harding and coworkers. However, their experiments were performed without defined extracellular calcium concentration. They report from a „maximum calcium effect", which they received within a range of 6-20 mM extracellular calcium [10,11].

Beuckelmann et al. examined the calcium homeostasis in isolated cardiomyocytes of non-failing and end-stage failing human hearts by means of the calcium indicator FURA-2. The action potential was found to be significantly prolonged in myocytes from end-stage failing hearts compared to non-failing hearts. In addition, a decreased ascent, a decreased amplitude and a delayed drop of intracellular calcium concentration was shown [9].

7.3.2. Influence of β-adrenoceptor agonists

We performed experiments with isoproterenol in order to examine the response of isolated cardiomyocytes from end-stage failing human hearts to β-adrenoceptor agonists. A dose-dependent increase in fractional shortening from 3.3±0,3 μm up to 7.9±1.4 μm (239 %) at a concentration of 10^{-7} M isoproterenol could be observed (Figure 6).

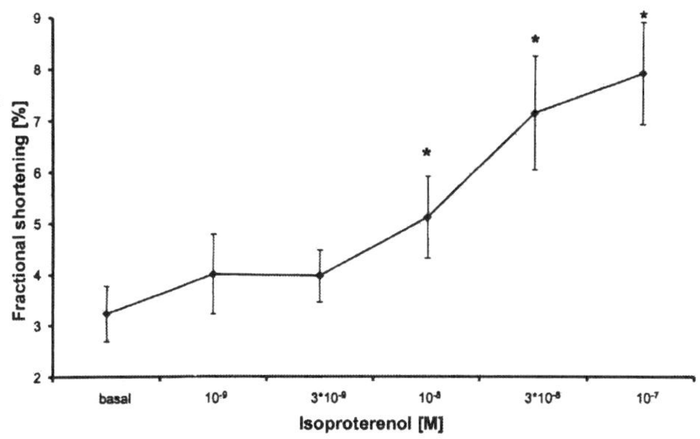

Figure 6: Fractional shortening [%] as a function of isoproterenol concentration [M]. Increase in fractional shortening is almost threefold at the highest isoproterenol concentration.

All contraction parameters showed significant changes indicating a shortened contraction.

Harding et al. could show an even more pronounced response to isoproterenol. High concentrations (exact values are not given) led to a fractional shortening of 10.4 %. Beside these findings, they compared the effects of isoproterenol on myocytes from non-failing and end-stage failing human hearts. A significant decrease concerning the response to isoproterenol in failing cardiomyocytes could be shown [12].

7.3.3. Post-rest contraction behaviour

Post-rest contractions show changes in fractional shortening of the first contraction after increasing rest intervals and are thougth to reflect the amount of calcium stored in and released from the sarcoplasmic reticulum [13]. By this non-invasive method changes of diastolic and systolic calcium concentrations are functionally detected. Normally rest periods from 10 s up to several minutes are examined in isolated cardiomyocytes. All data of post-rest contractions reported below are obtained from left ventricular myocytes.

Post-rest behaviour at low extracellular calcium (1.25 mM Ca^{2+})

In cells which were obtained from end-stage failing hearts, a fractional cell shortening of 3.7±0.3 % at basal stimulation rate (0.2 Hz) could be observed. With longer rest intervals, there was a continuous increase in fractional shortening at low extracellular calcium concentration [1.25 mM]. An increase of 140±6 % at 300 s rest from basal of 3.7±0.3 % to 5.2±0.6 % could be documented (Figure 7).

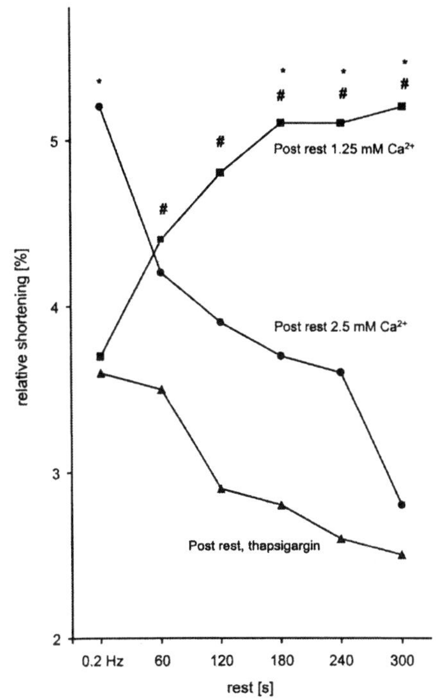

Figure 7: Post-rest experiments in left ventricular failing cardiomyocytes: At low calcium (1.25 mM) relative shortening increases with rest duration. At higher calcium (2.5 mM) relative shortening decreases with rest duration. After incubation with thapsigargin which blocks SR calcium ATPase relative shortening decreases with rest duration (see text).

In addition, velocities of shortening and relaxation as well as duration of contraction were inreased with longer rest intervals. However, at identical conditions post-rest potentiation in non-failing cardiomyocytes was even more pronounced: an increase of fractional shortening to 191±8 % (vs. 140±6 % in failing myocytes) could be detected (basal fractional shortening 2.3±1.0 %, at 300 s rest duration 4.4±1.8 %, Figure 8).

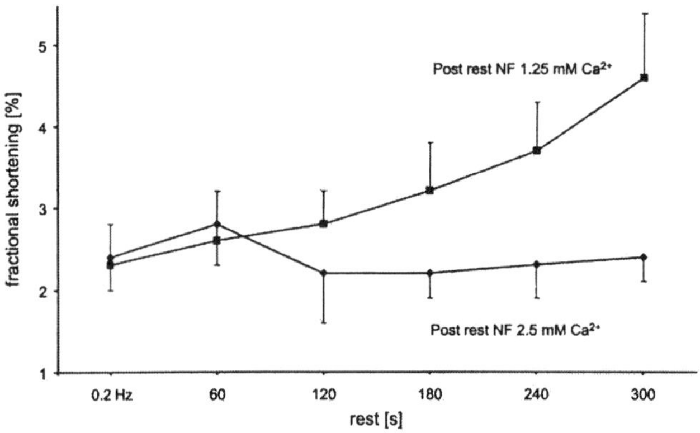

Figure 8: Post-rest experiments in left ventricular non-failing cardiomyocytes: At low calcium (1.25 mM) relative shortening increases with rest duration. At higher calcium (2.5 mM) relative shortening does not change significantly with rest duration (see text).

Post-rest behaviour at high extracellular calcium (2.5 mM Ca^{2+})

In failing cardiomyocytes baseline shortening at 0.2 Hz was 5.2±0.7 % at high extracellular Ca^{2+} concentrations [2.5 mM]. With increasing rest intervals, a continuous decrease of fractional shortening to 2.8±0.4 % at 300 s rest could be observed (Figure 7). This resulted in a post-rest decay of 58.8±3.7 %. Identical conditions (2.5 mM Ca^{2+}) did not significantly change post-rest behaviour in non-failing cardiomyocytes: Baseline values of 2.4±0.6 % at 0.2 Hz were measured. After 300 s rest there was no difference in fractional shortening detectable (2.6±0.3 %, Figure 8).

Davia et al. showed controverse results: In experiments performed with failing cardiomyocytes with high extracellular calcium (4-8 mM), they found a post-rest contraction without the decay mentioned above. Moreover, their experiments with non-failing cardiomyocytes even resulted in an inverse post-rest relationship [14].

7.3.4. Effects of thapsigargin on SR

Thapsigargin is able to block the pumping function of SR Calcium ATPase [15]. In myocytes from failing hearts we found depressed post-rest contractions even at low calcium concentrations after inactivation of the SR function by thapsigargin [10^{-6} M]. After 300 s rest a total decay of 29.2±3.6 % vs. baseline shortening of 3.6±0.6 % could be observed (Figure 7). Because of limited numbers of donor hearts, no experiments could be performed with non-failing cells concerning the effects of thapsigargin.
Our results are in good correspondance to experiments performed by Davia et al. [14]. They also found an inverse post-rest relationship in failing cardiomyocytes after preincubation with thapsigargin.

7.3.5. Force-frequency relationship

Bowditch and Blinks were the first to describe a positive inotropic effect triggered by an increasing heart rate. They performed experiments with a whole frog heart and muscle strip preparations, respectively [16,17]. To investigate these effects on the cellular level, we performed experiments with atrial and ventricular cardiomyocytes from failing and non-failing human hearts.
In ventricular myocytes from non-failing hearts, we could observe an increase of fractional shortening to 204 % with higher stimulation frequencies (1.7±0.4 % at 0.2 Hz to 3.5±0.8 % at 1.5 Hz, Figure 9). Myocytes isolated from right atria of non-failing hearts showed a positive force-frequency relationship as well. The increase was less pronounced than in non-failing ventricular myocytes (to 136 %, Figure 9).

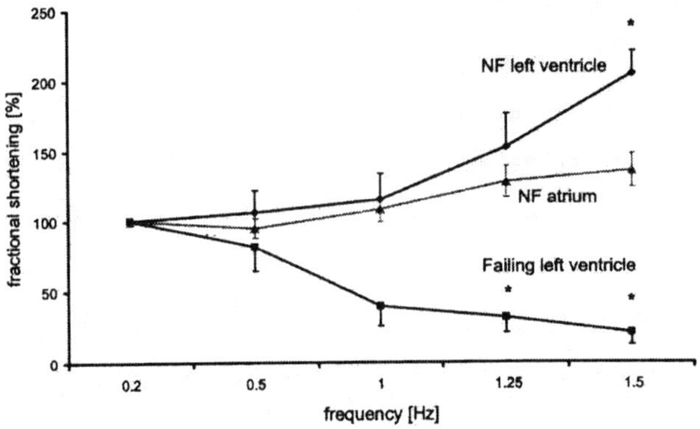

Figure 9: Force-frequency relationships in isolated cardiomyocytes: Positive force-frequency relationships are observed in nonfailing (NF) left ventricular and nonfailing right atrial cardiomyocytes. In contrast, an inverse force-frequency relationship is found in failing left ventricular cardiomyocytes.

However, in failing cardiomyocytes increasing stimulation frequencies (0.2 Hz up to 1.5 Hz) resulted in a significant decline of fractional shortening from 3.8±0.3 % to 0.8±0.2 % (Figure 9). Thereby, a negative force-frequency with a decay of 74 % resulted. TTP and RT_{50} were significantly reduced.
Davies et al. found an abolished, not an inverse force-frequency relationship in failing cardiomyocytes. However, their experiments were performed using a higher extracellular calcium concentration (2 mM) than in ours (1.25 mM) and therefore can not directly be compared [18].

7.3.6. Influence of vasoactive peptides

The single cell method turned out to be very suitable to investigate potentially inotropic effects of different substances. Our group showed special interest in the vasoactive peptides angiotensin II and endothelin-1. In addition to investigate the inotropic effects, experiments were performed in order to examine the intracellular signaling pathway.

7.3.6.1. Angiotensin II

We showed that angiotensin II has significant effects on contractile performance in isolated cardiomyocytes of human atrial tissue. As shown in Figure 10, the extent and velocity of shortening as well as the duration of contraction were profoundly increased.

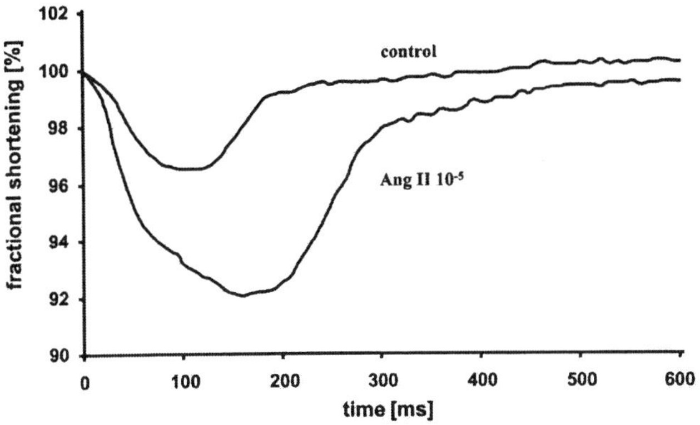

Figure 10: Effect of angiotensin II on isolated right atrial cardiomyocytes: typical records are shown for control and angiotensin II (Ang II, 10^{-5} maximum effect).

On the average, the extent of shortening was approximately doubled by angiotensin concentrations greater than 10^{-7} M (Figure 11).

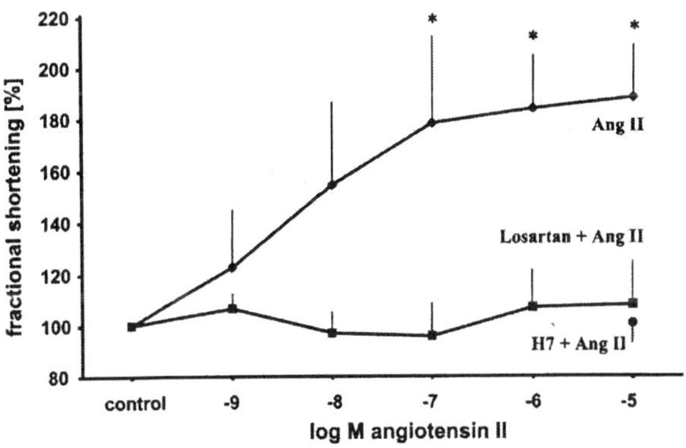

Figure 11: Dose-response curves for angiotensin II (Ang II) in right atrial cardiomyocytes: Note the dose-dependent increase in fractional shortening. The specific angiotensin-subtype 1-receptor antagonist losartan completely blocked this effect as well as H7, an inhibitor of proteinkinase C.

This effect on shortening extent was dose-dependent and could be completely blocked by previous application of the specific angiotensin-subtype 1-receptor-antagonist losartan (Figure 11). Moreover, angiotensin II did not exert any positive inotropic effects after preincubation with the proteinkinase C inhibitor H7 as well [19]. In contrast to these results, Lefroy et al. could not find any effect by angiotensin II in human cardiomyocytes at all [20].
Regarding ventricular myocytes their results are in good agreement with ours: angiotensin II, in all concentrations used, had no effect on the contractility of cardiomyocytes isolated from failing or non-failing human left ventricles. After lowering the extracellular pH_o to 7.0, angiotensin II did neither influence contractility.

7.3.6.2. Endothelin-1

Endothelin-1 effects on atrial myocytes
Quantitatively, endothelin-1 showed almost the same effect on contractility of atrial human cardiomyocytes as angiotensin II. 10^{-8} M endothelin-1 had this profound effect on the extent of fractional cell shortening as shown in Figure 12.

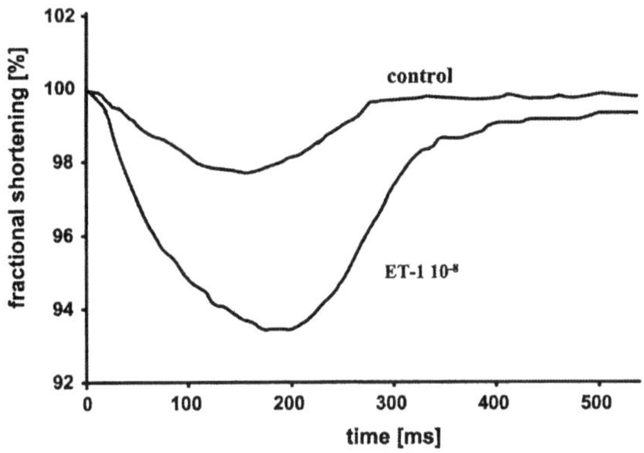

Figure 12: Effect of endothelin-1 (10^{-8} M) on right atrial human cardiomyocytes: Endothelin-1 (ET-1) profoundly increases extent of shortening as well as shortening and relaxation time.

There was a significant increase in velocities of cell shortening and relaxation, whereas the absolute time to peak shortening and the time to half-maximum relaxation did not differ significantly from control measurements. This positive inotropic effect was dose-dependent and could be blocked by the endothelin subtype A receptor antagonist BQ 123 (Figure 13).

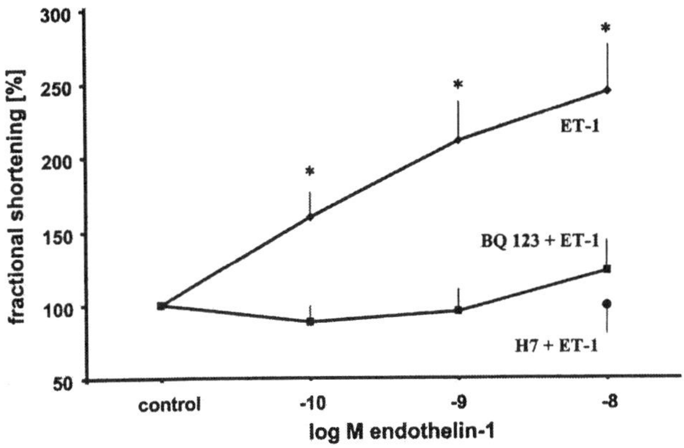

Figure 13: Dose-response curves for endothelin-1 (ET-1) in right atrial human cardiomyocytes: This effect was completely blocked by addition of the endothelin-subtype A-receptor antagonist BQ 123 as well as incubation with H7, an inhibitor of proteinkinase C.

On the average, the extent of shortening was more than doubled at higher concentrations ($\geq 10^{-9}$ M). In contrast to angiotensin II, however, the concentration needed to exert equipotent effects was about one hundred times lower for endothelin-1 (comparison of Figures 10 and 12).
Endothelin-1 was proposed to activate the sodium hydrogen exchanger (NHE) resulting in an intracellular alkalosis [21,22]. The calcium responsiveness of myofilaments critically depends on intracellular pH_i [23]. Therefore we tested the effects of endothelin after inhibition of the NHE with amiloride (10^{-5} M). This intervention did not influence the positive inotropic properties of endothelin-1. However, endothelin-1 lost the positive effect on the contractility after preincubation with the proteinkinase C inhibitor H7 (10^{-7} M, Figure 13).

Endothelin-1 effects on ventricular myocytes

In non-failing human left ventricular cardiomyocytes, endothelin-1 showed significant effects (+102 %) on the extent of shortening . This effect was dose-dependent and fractional shortening increased from 3.1±0.5 % on basal conditions to 6.2±1.7 % when endothelin (10^{-8} M) was added (Figure 14). There was a non-significant reduction in the time to peak shortening and time to half-maximum relaxation.

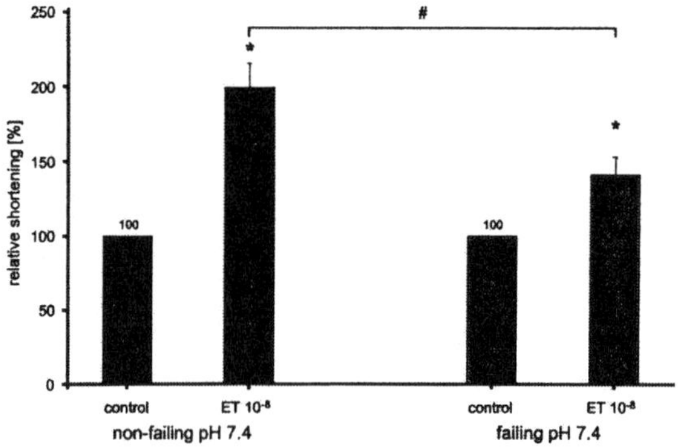

Figure 14: Effect of endothelin-1 (ET-1, 10^{-8} M) in nonfailing human left ventricular cardiomyocytes ***(left)*** *and on failing human left ventricular cardiomyocytes* ***(right)****. In failing human myocytes, the profound positive inotropic effect of endothelin-1 is markedly attenuated.*

Endothelin-1 showed a positive effect (+41 %) on the contractility of cardiomyocytes isolated from failing human hearts as well (fractional shortening basal 4.6±1.0 %, endothelin-1 (10^{-8} M) 6.6±1.1 %). However, this effect was significantly reduced compared to myocytes from non-failing hearts (Figure 14). Concerning the endothelin-1 results, no significant difference could be found between myocytes obtained from ischemic heart disease and those obtained from dilative heart disease (no Figure).

There is evidence for endothelin to increase the intracellular pH as mentioned above [21]. We therefore investigated the effects of endothelin in the presence of extracellular acidosis. The reduction of extracellular pH (pH_o) to 7.0 had the following effects: (1) Relative shortening was reduced to 83±3 % of the basal value at pH_o 7.4. (2) The time parameters were unchanged by this intervention. If failing cardiomyocytes were made acidic, endothelin showed a pronounced positive inotropic effect in failing myocardium as well: In acidic myocytes (pH_o 7.0) 10^{-8} M endothelin-1 more than doubled fractional shortening as well as velocities of shortening and relaxation (Figure 15). Time to peak shortening and time to half-maximum relaxation showed a small non-significant decrease that is similar to our findings in non-failing cardiomyocytes.

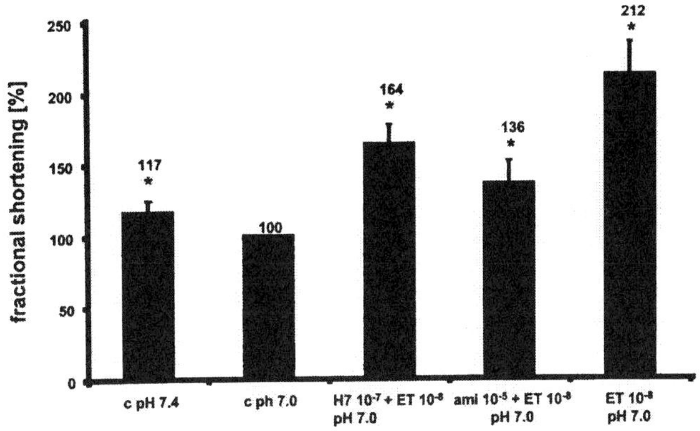

Figure 15: Effect of endothelin-1 (ET-1) on failing human left ventricular cardiomyocytes at low pH. There is a profound positive inotropic effect of ET-1 (right column). This effect is partially diminished by preincubation with amiloride, an inhibitor of the sodium-hydrogen-exchanger, and partially by addition of H7, an inhibitor of proteinkinase C.

This strong inotropic effect observed at a pH_0 of 7.0 could partially be blocked by 5-(N,N-dimethyl)-amiloride, a selective inhibitor of the NHE (10^{-5} M). Preincubation with amiloride reduced the positive inotropic properties of endothelin at extracellular acidosis from +112 % to only +35 % as compared to control (Figure 15). After inhibition of the proteinkinase C with H7, the endothelin-1 effect in acidic cells was also diminished to +64 % as compared to control (Figure 15).

7.4. Discussion

7.4.1. Discussion of Methods

There are different methods for research on contractile performance of the heart. A lot of parameters can be evaluated in vivo: cardiac index, left ventricular ejection fraction, stroke work index, to name but a few. However, preload and afterload as well as neuroendocrine reactions of the organism may influence all these parameters. To examine pure inotropic effects, examinations on isolated muscle preparations seem more reasonable.

For these purposes at least two different methods are available at the present time: muscle strip preparations (see Chapter III) and isolated cardiomyocytes. Experiments in muscle strip preparations can be performed on physiological conditions (temperature 37 °C, stimulation rate 1 Hz). However, it turned out that these conditions are not applicable to the single cell method. Therefore "slightly" unphysiological conditions (temperature 32 °C, stimulation rate 0.2 Hz) had to be chosen in order to get reproducable results. One important advantage of the single cell method is the possibility to rule out any influences of non-myocytes. In multicellular preparations, however, positive inotropic effects of substances that are to be evaluated may not be directly receptor-mediated. Left ventricular preparations either obtained from free left ventricular wall or from papillary muscles contain various non-myocyte cells: (1) In these preparations, small vessels and capillaries are present. In addition especially the endothelium may functionally influence the contractility of myocytes [24]. (2) Sympathetic nerve endings are predominantly found in atrial myocardium, but, to a lesser degree, also in ventricular myocardium. Norepinephrine may be released from these structures in an unpredictable way [25]. Furthermore, concentrations of substances needed to induce functional effects in multicellular preparations depend on diffusion distances and therefore do not reflect the true physiological effect on the cellular level. In addition, in muscle strip preparations the exact concentration of substances at the level of myocytes can only be estimated because of unforeseeable diffusion barriers. On the other hand, the single cell method assures defined concentrations without these diffusion barriers.

Some groups compared results of muscle strip preparations and isolated cardiomyocytes directly. Harding et al found that muscle strip preparations have advantages in measurement of force development, whereas other contractile parameters show smaller dispersion in single cell experiments [26]. However, results of single cell experiments and muscle strip preparations can be compared as has been shown by Weiser et al. [27].

In discussion with other researchers, there are some "frequently asked questions" concerning the single cell method: (1) Are the cells and the cell membranes intact after isolation? (2) Does longer transportation time of myocardial tissue influence the results? (3) Is the amount of fractional shortening on basal conditions comparable to the state of disease of the heart? (4) How is it possible to compare the inotropic effects in different cells? (5) Is the fact that single cells are contracting under isotonic conditions rather than under isometric important for the discussion of the results?

Ad (1): Enzymatic isolation of cardiomyocytes using the "chunk"-method, as described above, is a rather aggressive method. Cutting the tissues results in mechanical damage and in a massive calcium release to the myofilaments, which causes contractures. Enzymatic proteolysis could also affect the cell function. These limiting factors are represented in the yield of morphologically intact cells: only 10-30-(50) % of the cells fulfilled the requirements defined in the "Methods". However, these cells showed profound inotropic response to increasing extracellular calcium concentrations on the one hand and to β-adrenergic stimulation by isoproterenol on the other hand. These reproducible results indicate that cell membranes, sarcolemmal transport proteins, and receptors are intact in morphologically "healthy" cells after the isolation procedures.

Ad (2): The transportation time of myocardial tissues might influence the contractility of isolated cardiomyocytes. To diminish possible damage during transportation BDM was added to the tyrode solution. BDM was shown to save the myocardium from contractures caused by calcium release [6]. It has no significant influence on contractile behaviour after having been completely washed out [28]. Using this method, transportation or storage time up to 12 hours resulted in isolation of intact cardiomyocytes. Moreover, no differences could be found in experiments performed after short and long transportation time, respectively.

Ad (3): One could expect that cardiomyocytes isolated from non-failing myocardium show a larger extent in fractional shortening than cardiomyocytes originated from failing human hearts. However, our results do not correspond to this expectation: The average fractional shortening of non-failing cardiomyocytes on basal conditions was 3.0±0.7 %, whereas cells from end-stage human hearts showed an average shortening of 4.2±1.0 %. This evidence points to the fact that fractional shortening is not at all a parameter to differentiate between normal and failing isolated cells. For this purpose, the time parameters and diastolic cell length turned out to be more reliable: Time to peak contraction and time to half maximum relaxation were significantly shorter in non-failing cardiomyocytes compared to failing cardiomyocytes (TTP 435±81 ms versus 729±167 ms, $RT_{50\%}$ 713±159 ms versus 1243±223 ms). Gerdes et al. found significant differences in the diastolic length of isolated cardiomyocytes from non-failing and failing hearts [29]. Non-failing cardiomyocytes turned out to have the smallest diastolic length, whereas cells of hearts with ischemic cardiomyopathy were significantly longer. Cells originated from hearts with dilated cardiomyopathy showed the largest diastolic length [29,30].

Ad (4): For evaluation of single cell experiments, it is important to compare the relative change of fractional shortening. Contractions on basal conditions should be seen as a starting position (100%) and further contractions should be compared to this basal value. Thereby different experiments can be better related to each other.

Ad (5): Isolated myocytes contract under isotonic conditions. This fact is in contrast to the physiological contraction of the myocardium, which represents a combination between isotonic and isometric behaviour. However regarding contraction parameters it has been shown that there are no significant differences in measurements of isometric and isotonic contractions, respectively [31]. These results were obtained on muscle strip preparations, but they can be transferred to single cells in the most cases. One exception is mentioned in the next paragraph – increasing calcium concentrations lead to a continous decrease of the diastolic cell length and thereby to a loss of potentially inotropic properties.

7.4.2. Discussion of Results

7.4.2.1. Extracellular calcium

Increasing extracellular calcium concentrations lead to a higher transsarcolemmal calcium influx and thereby to a positive inotropic effect. We systematically examined the effects of different calcium concentrations on isolated cells. High calcium levels had a profound inotropic effect and, in addition, we found a significantly prolonged contraction (see Figures 4 and 5). The maximum inotropic effect at $[Ca^{2+}]_o$ 15 mM in isolated cells was 269 % vs. baseline conditions at $[Ca^{2+}]_o$ 1.25 mM, whereas muscle strip preparations showed an increase up to 427 % under identical conditions. This phenomenon might be explained by the fact that muscle strip preparations contract under constant isometric conditions, whereas single cells can change their diastolic length. The diastolic length depends, among other things, on the extracellular

calcium concentration and it decreases with increasing calcium concentration [9]. As mentioned above, the responsiveness to inotropic interventions decreases in this case because of unfavourable changes in the sarcomere length.
Results of Harding et al. indicate that there is no significant difference in the inotropic effect to calcium in cells from non-failing and failing human hearts, respectively [10,11].

7.4.2.2. Isoproterenol

Isoproterenol showed dose-dependent profound inotropic effects in isolated myocytes. Isoproterenol is a non-selective β-adrenoceptor agonist and increases the intracellular amount of cAMP by stimulation of the adenylatecyclase. Higher levels of cAMP cause an activation of proteinkinase A, which again is responsible for phosphorylation of different cellular proteins: phosphorylation of the L-type calcium channels leads to an increased calcium influx [32]. Phosphorylation of phospholamban reduces his inhibitory effect on the activity of the SR calcium ATPase, which leads to a higher calcium uptake in the SR [33].
In the failing human heart, the expression of β-adrenoceptors is significantly downregulated [34]. According to these data, the responsiveness of isolated cardiomyocytes from failing hearts was reduced in comparison to non-failing human hearts [12].

7.4.2.3. Post-rest relationship

In addition to the force-frequency relationship, the post-rest contraction of myocardium is thought to describe best the function of SR. The SR plays a major role in the calcium homeostasis. The calcium amount of the SR can be estimated with post-rest contractions as described by Ravens et al. [13]. During rest, calcium is stored from the cytosol into the SR by the SR calcium ATPase and removed to the extracellular space mainly by the Na^+/Ca^{2+} exchanger [35,36]. Calcium leaking from the SR can either be taken back by the SR or it can get lost from the cytosol through the Na^+/Ca^{2+} exchanger. Therefore, during rest calcium content might either increase, stay equal or decline in reliance of activity of the competitive pumps (SR calcium ATPase vs. Na^+/Ca^{2+} exchanger). Thereby, post-rest contractions may be potentiated or diminished.

Our results indicate (1) a post-rest potentiation at low extracellular calcium [1.25mM] in failing as well as in non-failing human cardiomyocytes. (2) In

contrast, a rest decay could be found in failing cardiomyocytes with increasing rest intervals at higher extracellular calcium [2.5mM]. In non-failing cardiomyocytes post-rest contraction stayed equal with this calcium concentration. (3) Inactivating SR function by thapsigargin abolished post-rest potentiation even at low extracellular calcium in failing cardiomyocytes.
These results are in good agreement to those of Pieske et al. who worked on similar conditions with muscle strip preparations. They could find a well preserved post-rest potentiation in muscle strips of non-failing hearts and a significant decay of post-rest contraction in muscle strips of end-stage failing hearts [37]. However, results of Davia et al. obtained from experiments performed with isolated single cells do not correspond to our findings [14]. They showed a decline in post-rest contraction in cells of non-failing hearts. This post-rest decrease was even more pronounced than in cells of end-stage failing hearts. However, their experiments were performed with changing and unphysiological extracellular calcium levels (4-8mM).

Our results indicate that post-rest behaviour critically depends on extracellular calcium levels. In cells of non-failing hearts, post-rest contractions were only positive at low extracellular calcium levels [1.25mM]. There was no change in fractional shortening of post rest contractions in experiments performed at higher extracellular calcium levels [2.5 mM]. This phenomenon might be explained by the regulation of Na^+/Ca^{2+} exchanger. Higher extracellular calcium levels correspond with higher intracellular calcium levels. The Na^+/Ca^{2+} exchanger is reported to get activated with increasing extracellular calcium levels [38]. Thereby the Na^+/Ca^{2+} exchanger is competing for intracellular calcium with the SR calcium ATPase. This situation results in a loss of calcium from intracellular storage compartments by an overactivity of the Na^+/Ca^{2+} exchanger in correspondance to the activity of the SR calcium ATPase, and thereby in an impaired post-rest contraction.

Different groups found a depressed expression of the SR calcium ATPase and an upregulation of the Na^+/Ca^{2+} exchanger in the failing heart [39-41]. Our results obtained from cardiomyocytes from end-stage failing hearts reflect this situation. Whereas in myocytes from non-failing hearts the post-rest contraction was doubled after 300 s at low extracellular calcium, there was only an increase of 40 % detectable in failing cardiomyocytes on identical conditions. We even found a negative post-rest contraction at higher extracellular calcium levels in myocytes of failing hearts. This indicates the relative predominance of the Na^+/Ca^{2+} exchanger vs. the SR calcium ATPase in cardiomyocytes of failing hearts, which results in decreased intracellular calcium levels and thereby in a decreased contractility. By blocking the function of the SR this situation even gets worse: the cell is disabled to store calcium in intracellular compartments. At the same time, there is a continuous loss of calcium through the Na^+/Ca^{2+} exchanger, especially at longer rest (diastolic) periods, which results in a negative post-rest contraction even at low extracellular calcium levels.

7.4.2.4. Force-frequency relationship

It is known for a long time that force development in mammalian hearts increases with higher stimulation frequencies [42]. This result could be confirmed for non-failing human muscle in vitro and in vivo [43,44]. However, this positive force-frequency relationship was neutralized [18] or even reversed in preparations of end-stage failing human hearts [44]. Since it could not be excluded that fibrosis or other changes of the extracellular matrix in failing human myocardium contribute to this phenomenon, we performed experiments with isolated cells [45].

Whereas left ventricular cells from non-failing hearts showed a pronounced positive force-frequency relationship, cells from failing human hearts showed an reversed force-frequency relationship. These results are in excellent agreement with those of Pieske et al. who performed their experiments with muscle strip preparations [44]. In addition, the force-frequency relationship in atrial cells of non-failing hearts was positive, even though to a lesser degree than left ventricular cells (Figure 9).

However, results of Davies et al. do not correspond exactly to ours: They could show a neutralized, not a reversed force-frequency response in isolated cells from failing human hearts. Again, these experiments were performed with a higher extracellular calcium concentration [2 mM].

Some groups found a reduced amount of activating calcium in left ventricular preparations of failing human hearts at higher stimulation frequencies, which could contribute to the decreased frequency response [44,46]. As described above, alterations in gene expression of the SR calcium ATPase and the Na^+/Ca^{2+} exchanger could be responsible for this phenomenon. The intact ratio of these two transport proteins in non-failing hearts leads to an increased calcium storage in the SR with increasing frequencies resulting in a positive force-frequency relationship. However, in failing human hearts, the Na^+/Ca^{2+} exchanger is relatively predominant compared to the SR calcium ATPase. This reverse ratio results in a continuous decline of stored calcium, which leads to diminished contractions especially at higher stimulation frequencies.

Clinical relevance

Experiments performed in vivo showed an inverse force-frequency relationship in patients with end-stage heart failure [43,47]. This finding is in excellent agreement with those of single cell or muscle strip experiments in vitro. It indicates that rather changes on the level of cardiomyocytes are responsible for this phenomenon than extramyocardial changes. In addition, these results partly explain the beneficial effects of current therapeutic strategies in heart failure: By decreasing the heart rate, β-adrenoceptor blockers may directly attenuate the force-frequency abnormality in patients with an inverted relationship. This provides myocardial calcium cycling proteins with more time to achieve calcium homeostasis and the sarcoplasmic reticulum adequate time to reprime itself. Both, digitalis glycosides and ACE inhibitors reduce adrenergic stimulation and thus secondarily favorably influence the inverted force-frequency relationship by slowing heart rate. ACE inhibitors may also have other effects that directly reverse the underlying abnormalities in calcium pumping [48].

In addition, these results as well as the results of post-rest contractions mentioned above elucidate the functional consequences of altered gene expression in failing human hearts on the level of isolated single myocytes.

7.4.2.5. Vasoactive peptides

Oligopeptides like angiotensin II and endothelin-1 are biologically and pathophysiologically important, because they do not only regulate vascular tone and thereby blood pressure. They also may contribute to the regulation of myocardial contractility. Both oligopeptides may function as a hormonal coupling system between the endothelium where they are generated and released and the myocardium where they bind to their specific receptors.

Endothelin-1 has been shown to elicit pronounced positive inotropic effects in rabbit myocardium, moderate action in guinea pig and rat myocardium, but it had no influence on myocardial contractility in isolated dog myocardium [49]. Since endothelin-1 plasma levels [50] and myocardial endothelin-1-receptor densities were found to be elevated in dilative cardiomyopathy [51,52], we investigated the effects of endothelin-1 in isolated cardiomyocytes from non-failing and end-stage failing human hearts.

A number of studies [53,54] has identified the existence of all components of a local renin-angiotensin system in the myocardium including angiotensin II receptors [55]. Such a local autocrine or paracrine system may have short-term function, i. e., regulation of myocardial contractility as well as long-term effects, i. e., stimulation of myocardial growth [56]. We therefore investigated the effects of angiotensin II on isolated myocytes thereby excluding any possible effects of non-myocyte components. In addition, we investigated the subcellular signaling pathway of the angiotensin II response.

Angiotensin II in atrial human myocardium

In single cardiac myocytes isolated from human atria we found a dose-dependent cardiotonic effect of angiotensin II. This finding is in good agreement with previous work on muscle strip preparations done by our group [28] and others [57]. This effect is clearly subtype-1 angiotensin-receptor mediated, because it can be blocked by losartan. In muscle strip preparations loaded with the calcium-indicator aequorin, this cardiotonic effect of angiotensin was associated with an increase in calcium transients [58].

Angiotensin II is known to activate the phosphatidylinositol-4,5-biphosphate pathway thereby increasing both proteinkinase C (PKC) via diacylglycerol (DG) and inositol-1,4,5-triphosphate (IP_3). Because we have shown that the angiotensin II induced positive inotropic response is blocked by the selective PKC-inhibitor H7, we can conclude that phosphorylation of either phospholamban, sarcoplasmic reticulum ATPase or sarcolemmal calcium channels (or all of them) mediates this inotropic effect.

Endothelin-1 in atrial human myocardium

We could demonstrate a profound and significant influence of endothelin-1 on the contractility of human atrial cardiomyocytes. Quantitatively, this effect is similar to that of angiotensin, however reached at much lower concentrations (comparison of Figure 10 with Figure 12). Therefore, the endothelin-1-induced effect may be of greater physiological relevance. This inotropic effect is shown to be endothelin-receptor mediated, because it was completely blocked by the selective ET_A-receptor blocker BQ 123 (Figure 13). Meyer et al [22] have demonstrated significant inotropic properties of endothelin 1 in trabecular preparations of human atria, although the increase in force development was only about 30 %, whereas the increase in the extent of shortening is about 150 % in our study.

As with angiotensin II, these authors demonstrated that the positive inotropic effect of endothelin is associated with a similar increase of the intracellular calcium transient. Similar to the findings with angiotensin II, the endothelin-1 effects were blunted after preincubation with the protein kinase C inhibitor H7. Therefore, endothelin-1 seems to have the same subcellular signaling pathway in atrial cardiomyocytes as described for angiotensin II (see above).

Angiotensin II in left ventricular human myocardium

We could not find any effect of angiotensin II on cardiomyocytes of left ventricular human myocardium despite a well-preserved contractile reserve as demonstrated by application of isoproterenol (10^{-7} M) or high extracellular calcium levels (15 mM). These results are in excellent agreement with those of Lefroy et al [20] who also used isolated human myocytes as well as with our own data obtained in left ventricular human muscle strips [28]. Interestingly, Moravec et al. reported on a positive inotropic effect of angiotensin II [57]. However, this effect could be found only in one third of their muscle strip preparations from left ventricular human myocardium (on non-physiological conditions).

Endothelin-1 in left ventricular human myocardium

Endothelin-1 showed a significant positive inotropic effect in isolated human cardiomyocytes of non-failing hearts (+99 %). This positive inotropic effect was significantly diminished to +41 % in cardiomyocytes of end-stage failing myocardium. Moravec [59] observed a very small positive inotropic effect in muscle strips of failing human hearts (+9 %). Suzuki showed an altered and decreased inotropic response to endothelin in failing compared to non-failing rat hearts [60].

Our results are for the most part in correspondence with findings of Pieske et al [51]. These authors compared muscle strip preparations from failing and non-failing human myocardium regarding the positive inotropic effect of endothelin-1. In failing myocardium the effect of endothelin-1 was also less pronounced than in non-failing myocardium (36 % vs. 52 %). This quantitative difference between isolated myocytes and muscle strip preparations may be explained by the assumption of a hypoxic and therefore acidic core in muscle strip preparations. At low pH endothelin-1 has a greater positive inotropic effect than at normal pH (see below).

A decrease in extracellular pH_o produces parallel changes in intracellular pH_i [61]. The calcium responsiveness of myofilaments critically depends on intracellular pH_i [23]. The decreased calcium sensitivity at low pH_i may be due to direct competition of hydrogen ions with calcium ions for a binding site on troponin C [62]. According to these data, we found a decrease of the extent of relative cell shortening after lowering the pH_o to 7.0 (Figure 15). Extracellular acidosis, however, increased the positive inotropic properties of endothelin (+112 % instead of +41 % at pH_o 7.4). Endothelin has been reported to stimulate transsarcolemmal H^+ extrusion by activation of the NHE resulting in intracellular alkalosis, which again leads to an improved responsiveness of myofilaments to calcium [21]. We therefore tested the effect of endothelin at

pH_o 7.0 after selectively blocking the NHE by means of amiloride. Under these circumstances endothelin exerted a similar effect as at physiological pH_0 of 7.4. The extent of relative cell shortening increased only by 36 %. In addition, we tested the effect of endothelin at pH_o 7.0 after preincubation with H7 as a selective proteinkinase C inhibitor. The positive inotropic property of endothelin was diminished to +64 % (Figure 15).

So, neither blocking of PKC nor blocking of NHE could completely abolish the effects of endothelin-1. It can be concluded that there must be other mechanisms on the level of the second messenger system than PKC as well as other mediators than NHE. These findings are in excellent correspondence to Krämer et al. [21]. These authors found an endothelin induced alkalosis mediated by activation of NHE. However they postulated other unknown mechanisms of the endothelin-effect.

Since endothelin receptors are not downregulated but rather upregulated in failing myocardium, the differences in endothelin-1-induced effects in non-failing and failing human myocardium can only be explained by the different regulation of second messenger systems and different mediators of inotropic action.

Clinical relevance

Plasma levels of angiotensin II are elevated in human heart failure leading to increased peripheral resistance via angiotensin II receptor stimulation of vascular smooth muscle cells. Use of angiotensin-converting-enzyme (ACE) inhibitors reduces preload and afterload and improves survival rate of patients with heart failure. Angiotensin II showed no inotropic effect in isolated ventricular myocytes and therefore ACE-inhibitor therapy does not reduce myocardial contractility.

The inotropic effects of endothelin-1 in human myocardium are ET_A-receptor-mediated. These receptors are also found on coronary arteries and peripheral vessels mediating vasoconstriction [63]. This leads to a decreased coronary blood flow as well as an increased afterload. Phosphoramidon, an endothelin-conversion-enzyme (ECE) inhibitor, has been shown to reduce infarct size in a model of myocardial ischemia and reperfusion in rats [64]. In addition, the specific ET_A receptor antagonist BQ-123 reduces infarct size after coronary occlusion and reperfusion in a canine model [65]. Short-term treatment of patients with severe chronic heart failure with the non-selective endothelin receptor antagonist bosentan resulted in beneficial acute hemodynamic effects with reduced systemic and pulmonary vascular resistance and increased cardiac output [66].

On the other hand, as above, endothelin significantly increases myocardial contractility especially on acidic conditions. Blocking the effects of endothelin therefore might have both beneficial effects in terms of reducing afterload, increasing coronary blood flow and reducing Ca^{2+} overload during reperfusion injury as well as negative effects in terms of directly reducing myocardial contractility, especially in ischemic and acidic states.

REFERENCES

1) Powell T, Sturridge M, Suvarna S, Terrar D, and Twist V: Intact individual heart cells isolated from human ventricular tissue. Br Med J 1981; 283:1013-1015

2) Bustamente O, Watanabe T, Murphy D, and McDonald T: Isolation of single atrial and ventricular cells from the human heart. CMA J 1982; 126:791-793

3) Mitra R and Morad M: A uniform enzymatic method for dissociation of myocytes from hearts and stomachs of vertebrates. Am J Physiol 1985;249:H1056-H1060

4) Isenberg G and Klockner U: Calcium tolerant ventricular myocytes prepared by incubation in a KB medium. Pfluegers Arch 1982;395:6-18

5) Bustamente O, Watanabe T, and McDonald T: Nonspecific Protease: a new approach to isolation of adult cardiocytes. Can J Physiol Pharmacol 1982;60:997-1002

6) Mulieri L, Hasenfuss G, Ittleman F, Blanchard E, and Alpert N: Protection of human left ventricular myocardium from cutting injury with 2,3-Butanedione Monoxime. Circ Res 1989;65:1441-1444

7) Schwinger R, Böhm M, Koch A, Morano I, Rüegg J, and Erdmann E: Inotropic effect of the cardioprotective agent 2,3-Butanedione-Monoxime. J Pharmacol 1993;269:778-786

8) Ito N, Kagaya Y, Weinberg E, Barry W, and Lorell B: Endothelin and Angiotensin II Stimulation of NHE is impaired in cardiac hypertrophy. J Clin Invest 1997;99:125-135

9) Beuckelmann D, Nähbauer M, and Erdmann E: Intracellular calcium handling in isolated ventricular myocytes from patients with terminal heart failure. Circulation 1992;85:1046-1055

10) Harding S, Jones M, O'Gara P, Monte del F, Vescovo G, and Poole-Wilson P: Isolated ventricular myocytes from failing and non-failing human heart: the relation of age and clinical status of the patients to isoproterenol response. J Mol Cell Card 1992;24:549-564

11) Monte del F, O'Gara P, Poole-Wilson P, Yucoub M, and Harding S: Cell geometry and contractile abnormalities of myocytes from failing human left ventricle. Cardiovasc Res 1995;30:281-290

12) Harding S, Jones M, O'Gara P, Vescovo G, and Poole-Wilson P: Reduced beta-agonist sensitivity in single atrial cells from failing human hearts. Am J Physiol 1990;259:H1009-H1014

13) Ravens U, Post-rest potentiation and its decay. In: The interval-force relationship in the heart. M. Nobled and W. Seed, Editors. 1993: Cambridge. pp 245-258

14) Davia K, Davies C, and Harding S: Effects of inhibition of sarcoplasmic reticulum calcium uptake on contraction in myocytes isolated from failing human ventricle. Cardiovasc Res 1997;33:88-97

15) Hakii H, Fujikii H, Suganuma M, Nakayasu M, Tahira T, Sugimura T, Scheurer P, and Christensen S: Thapsigargin, a histamine secretagogue, is a non-12-O-tetra-decanoylphorbol-13-acetate (TPA) type promotor in two-stage mouse skin carcinogenesis. Cancer Res Clin Oncol 1986;111:177-181

16) Bowditch H: Über die Eigentümlichkeiten der Reizbarkeit, welche die Muskelfasern des Herzens zeigen. Ber Sachs Ges (Akad) Wiss 1871;23:652-689

17) Blinks J and Koch-Weser J: Analysis of the effects of change in the rate and rythm upon myocardial contractility. J Pharmacol Exp The 1961;134:373-389

18) Davies C, Davia K, Bennett J, Peppe J, Poole-Wilson P, and Harding S: Reduced contraction and altered frequency response of isolated myocytes from patients with heart failure. Circulation 1995;92:2540-2549

19) Hidaka H, Inagaki M, Kawamoto S, and Sasaki Y: Isoquinolinesulfonamides, novel and potent inhibitors of cyclic nucleotide dependent protein kinase and protein kinase C. Biochem 1984;23:5036-5041

20) Lefroy D, Crale T, Monte del F, Vesecovo G, Liberia L, Harding S, and Poole-Wilson P: Angiotensin II and contraction of isolated myocytes from human, guinea pig and infarcted rat hearts. Am J Physiol 1996;270:H2060-H2069

21) Krämer B, Smith T, and Kelly R: Endothelin and increased contractility in adult rat ventricular myocytes. Role of intracellular alkalosis induced by activation of the protein kinase c-dependent NHE. Circ Res 1991;68:269-279

22) Meyer M, Lehnart S, Pieske B, Schlotthauer K, Munk S, Holubarsch C, Just H, and Hasenfuss G: Influence of endothelin-1 on human atrial myocardium - myocardial function and subcellular pathways. Bas Res Cardiol 1995;90:563-576

23) Allen D and Orchard C: The effects of changes of pH on intracellular calcium transients in mammalian myocardium. J Physiol 1983;335:555-567

24) Brutsaert D, Fransen P, Andries L, DeKeulenaer G, et al.: Cardiac endothelium and myocardial function. Cardiovasc Res 1998;38(2):281-290

25) Rump L, Schwertfeger E, Schaible U, Fraedrich G, and Schollmeyer P: Beta 2-adrenergic receptor and angiotensin II receptor modulation of sympathetic neurotransmission in human atria. Circ Res 1994;74:434-440

26) Harding S, Brown L, del Monte F, Davies C, O'Gara P, Vescovo G, Wynnw D, and Poole-Wilson P: Acceleration of contraction by beta-adrenoceptor stimulation is greater in ventricular myocytes from failing than non-failing human hearts. Bas Res Cardiol 1996;2:53-56

27) Weiser J, v. Lewinski D, Bisping E, Maier L, Janssen P, and Pieske B: Unterscheiden sich isolierte menschliche Herzmuskelzellen und Muskelstreifenpräparate in ihrem kontraktilen Verhalten? - Isometrische vs isotonische Verkürzung. Zeitschr Kard 1999;88 (suppl 1):787

28) Holubarsch C, Hasenfuss G, Schmidt-Schweda S, Knorr A, Pieske B, Ruf T, Fasol R, and Just H: Angiotensin I and II exerts inotropic effects in atrial but not in ventricular human

myocardium: An in vitro study under physiological experimental conditions. Circulation 1993;88:1228-1237

29) Gerdes A and Capasso J: Structural remodelling and mechanical dysfunction of cardiac myocytes in heart failure. J Mol Cell Cardiol 1995;27:849-856

30) Tamura T, Said S, Harris J, Lu W, and Gerdes A: Reverse remodeling of cardiac myocyte hypertrophy in Hypertension and failure by targeting of the renin-angiotensin system. Circulation 2000;102:253-259

31) Holubarsch C, Lüdemann J, Wiessner S, Ruf T, Schulte-Baukloh H, Schmidt-Schweda S, Pieske B, Posival H, and Just H: Shortening versus isometric contractions in isolated human failing and non-failing left ventricular myocardium: dependency of external work and force on muscle length, heart rate and inotropic stimulation. Cardiovasc Res 1998;37:46-57

32) Wohlfahrt B and Noble M: The cardiac excitation-contraction cycle. Pharmac Ther 1982;16:1-43

33) Movesian M, Karimi M, Green K, and Jones L: Calcium transporting, ATPAse, phospholamban, and calsequestrin levels in nonfailing and failing myocardium. Circulation 1994;90:653-657

34) Brodde O: Beta-1 and Beta-2-Adrenoceptors in the human heart: Properties, function, and alterations in chronic heart failure. Pharmacol Rev 1991;43:203-242

35) O'Neill S, Valdeolmillos M, Lamont C, Donoso P, and Eisner D: The contribution of natrium-calcium exchange to relaxation in mammalian cardiac muscle. Ann NY Acad Sci 1991;639:444-452

36) Bers D: Calcium influx and sarcoplasmatic reticulum calcium release in cardiac muscle activation during post-rest recovery. Am J Physiol 1985;248:H366-H381

37) Pieske B, Sütterlin M, Schmidt-Schweda S, Minami K, Meyer M, Olschewski M, Holubarsch C, Just H, and Hasenfuss G: Diminished post-rest potentiation of contractile force in human dilated cardiomyopathy. J Clin Invest 1996;98:764-776

38) Miura Y and Kimura J: Sodium-calcium exchange current: dependance on internal calcium and natrium and competitve binding of external calcium. J Gen Physiol 1989;93:1129-1145

39) Mercardier J, Lompre A, Due P, Boehler K, Fraysse J, Wisnewsky C, Allen P, Komjda M, and Schwartz K: Altered sarcoplasmic reticulum calcium ATPase gene expression in the human ventricle during endstage heart failure. J Clin Invest 1990;85:305-309

40) Hasenfuss G, Reinecke H, Studer R, Meyer M, Pieske B, Holtz J, Holubarsch C, Posival H, Just H, and Drexler H: Relation between myocardial function and expression of sarcoplasmic reticulum Calcium-ATPase in failing and nonfailing human myocardium. Circ Res 1994;75:434-442

41) Hasenfuss G, Schillinger W, Lehnart S, Preuss M, Pieske B, Maier L, Prestle J, Minami K, and Just H: Relationship between natrium-calcium exchanger protein levels and diastolic function of failing human myocardium. Circulation 1999;99:621-648

42) Koch-Weser J and Blinks J: The influence of the interval between beats on myocardial contractility. Pharmacol Rev 1963;15:601-652

43) Hasenfuss G, Holubarsch C, Hermann H, Astheimer K, Pieske B, and Just H: Influence of the force-frequency relationship on hemodynamics and left ventricular function in patients with non-failing hearts and in patients with dilated cardiomyopathy. Eur Heart J 1994;11645:170

44) Pieske B, Kretschmann B, Meyer M, Holubarsch C, Weirich J, Posival H, Minami K, Just H, and Hasenfuss G: Alterations in intracellular calcium handling associated with inverse force-frequency relation in human dilated cardiomyopathy. Circulation 1995;92:1169-1178

45) Weber K, Brilla C, and Janicki J: Myocardial fibrosis: functional significance and regulatory factors. Cardiovasc Res 1993;27:341-348

46) Sipido K, Stankovicoca T, Flameng W, Vanhaecke J, and Verdonk F: Frequency dependence of calcium release from the sarcoplasmic reticulum in human ventricular myocytes from end-stage heart failure. Cardiovasc Res 1998;37:478-488

47) Feldman A, Gwathmey J, Phillips P, Schoen F, and Morgan J: Reversal of the force-frequency relationship in working myocardium from patients with end-stage heart failure. J Appl Cardiol 1988;3:273-283

48) Holtz J, Studer R, Reinecke H, Just H, and Drexler H: Modulation of myocardial sarcoplasmic reticulum calcium ATPase in cardiac hypertrophy by angiotensin-converting enzyme? Bas Res Card 1992;87:191-204

49) Takanashi M and Endoh M: Characterization of positive inotropic effects of endothelin on mammalian ventricular myocardium. Am J Physiol 1991;261:H611-H619

50) Lerman A, Kubo S, Tschumperlin L, and Burnett J: Plasma endothelin concentrations in human with endstage heart failure and after heart transplantation. J Am Coll Card 1992;20:849-853

51) Pieske B, Beyermann B, Breu V, Löffler B, Schlotthauer K, Maier L, Schmidt-Schweda S, Just H, and Hasenfuss G: Functional effects of endothelin and regulation of endothelin receptors in isolated human nonfailing and failing myocardium. Circulation 1999;99:1802-1809

52) Pönicke K, Vogelsang M, Heinroth M, Becker K, Zolk O, Böhm M, Zerkowski H, and Brodde O: Endothelin receptors in the failing and nonfailing human heart. Circulation 1998;97:744-751

53) Schunkert H, Dzau V, Tang S, Hirsch A, Apstein C, and Lorell B: Increased cardiac angiotensin converting enzyme activity and mRNA expression in pressure overload left ventricular hypertrophy. J Clin Invest 1990;86:1913-1920

54) Lindpainter K, Jin M, Wilhelm M, Suzuki F, Linz W, Schoelkens B, and Ganten D: Intracardiac generation of angiotensin and its physiologic role. Circulation 1988;77:1-18

55) Regitz-Zagrosek V, Friedel N, Heymann A, and et al.: Regulation, chamber localization, and subtype distribution of angiotensin II receptors in human hearts. Circulation 1995;91:1461-1471

56) Lindpainter K and Ganten Ds:The cardiac renin-angiotensin system. Circ Res 1991;68:905-921

57) Moravec C, Schluchter M, Paranaudi L, Czerska B, Stewart R, Rosenkranz E, and Bond M: Inotropic effects of angiotensin II on human cardiac muscle in vitro. Circulation 1990;82:1973-1984

58) Holubarsch C, Pieske B, Kretschmann B, Schmidt-Schweda S, Meyer M, Schlotthauer K, Ruf T, Hasenfuss G, and Just H: The functional role of angiotensin II and endothelin-1 in the failing and nonfailing human myocardium. In: The Failing Heart. N. Dhalla, Editor. 1995, Raven Press: New York. pp 295-304

59) Moravec C, Reynolds E, Stewart R, and Bond M: Endothelin is a positive inotropic agent in human and rat heart in vitro. Biochem Biophys Res Commun 1989;159:14-18

60) Suzuki M, Nobuyuki O, Wang Z, Williams D, Little W, and Cheng C: Altered inotropic response of endothelin-1 in cardiomyocytes from rats with isoproterenol-induced cardiomyopathy. Cardiovas Res 1998;39:589-599

61) Fabiato A and Fabiato F: Effects of pH in the myofilaments and the sarcoplasmic reticulum of skinned cells from cardiac and skeletal muscles. J Physiol (Lond) 1978;276:233-255

62) Fuchs F, Reddy Y, and Briggs F: The interaction of cations with the calcium binding site of troponin. Biochem Biophys Acta 1970;221:407-409

63) Ihara M, Noguchi K, Saeki T, Fukuroda T, Tsuchida S, Kimura S, Fukami T, Ishikawa K, Nishikibe M, and Yano M: Biological profiles of highly potent novel endothelin antagonists selective for the ET A-receptor. Life Science 1991;50:247-255

64) Grover G, Sleph P, Fox M, and Trippodo N: Role of endothelin-1 and big endothelin-1 in modulating coronary vascular tone, contractile function and severity of ischemia in rat hearts. J Pharma & Exp Th 1992;263:1074-1082

65) Grover G, Dzwonczyk S, and Parham C: The endothelin-1 receptor antagonist BQ-123 reduces infarct size in a canine model of coronary occlusion and reperfusion. Cardiovasc Res 1993;27:1613-1618

66) Kiowski W, Sütsch G, Hunziker P, Müller P, Kim J, Oechslin E, Schmitt R, Jones R, and Bertel C: Evidence for endothelin-1-mediated vasoconstriction in severe chronic heart failure. Lancet 1995;346:732-736

8. DIASTOLIC COMPLIANCE

8.1. Introduction

Most of the patients reporting on typical symptoms of chronic heart failure suffer from left ventricular systolic dysfunction, i.e., present with a severely – or at least moderately – reduced left ventricular ejection fraction. However, about 10-30 % of these symptomatic patients have a normal left ventricular ejection fraction but signs of left ventricular concentric hypertrophy. Using modern clinical echocardiography, indirect indices of diastolic compliance disturbances may be found (for example a change in E/A ratio).

However, the concept of diastolic compliance heart failure has been established long before echocardiography had been developed for clinical purposes: Initially, alterations of left ventricular compliance have been attributed to simply geometrical factors, i.e., increased left ventricular muscle mass (Figure 1).

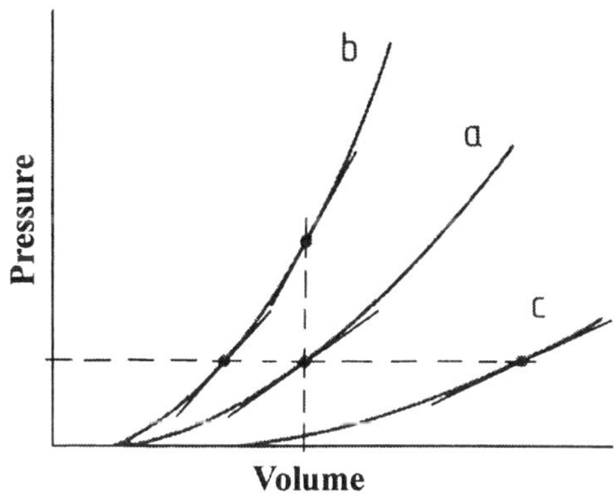

*Figure 1: Pressure-volume relationships of a normal left ventricle **(a)**, concentrically hypertrophied left ventricle (increased wall thickness, **(b)**, and excentrically hypertrophied left ventricle (dilatation, **(c)**).*

However, it became evident that the myocardium itself may be altered so that myocardial distensibility is decreased. Evaluation of this myocardial compliance in the whole heart or even in vivo has been attempted by the development of very complex mathematical equations taking into account the geometry and thickness of the left ventricle [1,2].

In animal models of cardiac hypertrophy and failure, myocardial compliance can be directly evaluated from the resting length-tension curve obtained from a longitudinal preparation of the right or left ventricle (see Methods of this chapter and also Chapter III). These experiments also allow microscopic and biochemical analysis of interstitial space of the myocardium (interstitial fibrosis). Another reason for disturbances of diastolic function of the myocardium may be impaired relaxation in the phase of late systole in hypertrophied and failing myocardium. Since impaired relaxation is due to alterations in calcium handling, heart rate dependency has to be considered implicating investigations at different low, medium, and high stimulation rates.

8.2. Methods

When a muscle strip preparation is stretched stepwise using 0.1 or 0.05 mm steps, the force imposed on the muscle is measured. From the change in muscle length Δl and the change in force ΔF, the passive length-tension curve of a specific muscle preparation is obtained. To allow comparisons between individual muscle preparations with different lengths and different cross-sectional areas (muscle diameters), force and length of the preparation must be normalized:

$$Strain\ \Delta\varepsilon = \frac{\Delta l}{l_o}$$

when strain Δε is the relative length change, Δl is the length change and l_0 is the length of muscle with no passive force, and

$$stress\ \Delta\sigma = \frac{\Delta F}{A}$$

when stress Δσ is the change in stress, ΔF is the change in force and A is the cross-sectional area (see Figure 2).

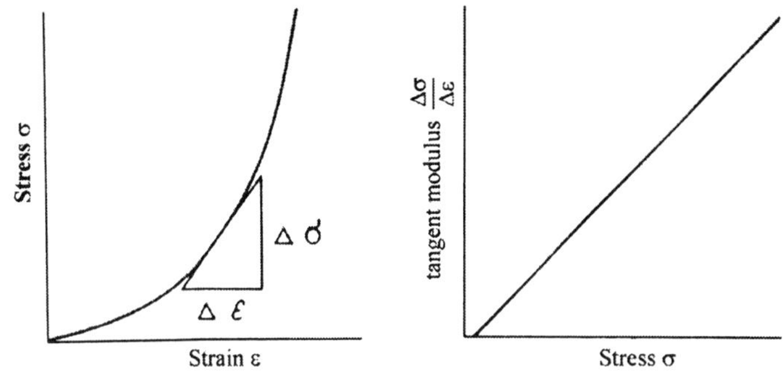

*Figure 2: Stress-strain relationship (**left**) and tangent modulus- stress relationship (**right**). The slope of the tangent modulus-stress relationship indicates myocardial stiffness.*

$E = \Delta\sigma/\Delta\varepsilon$ is the tangent elastic modulus, which can be plotted as a function of stress σ yielding a linear relationship (see Figure 2).
The slope of this function is the physical parameter which quantitatively defines myocardial stiffness.

Using complex equations and making certain assumptions regarding chamber geometry and stress distribution, the tangent elastic modulus may also be derived from whole heart measurement [1,2].

8.3. Results

8.3.1. Stress-Strain Rclationships in Isolated Muscle Strip Preparations

Several authors have demonstrated increased stiffness of the myocardium due to hypertrophy and failure in a variety of animal studies. Resting length-tension diagrams were shifted upwards and to the left (stiffer myocardium) in a cat model of right ventricular hypertrophy and failure [3,4], in a rat model of left ventricular hypertrophy [5], and in a rabbit model of right ventricular hypertrophy [6].

We have studied myocardial diastolic compliance in three models of cardiac hypertrophy in the rat: Despite huge increases of muscle mass due to thyrotoxicosis, myocardial stiffness was unchanged (Figure 3) [7].

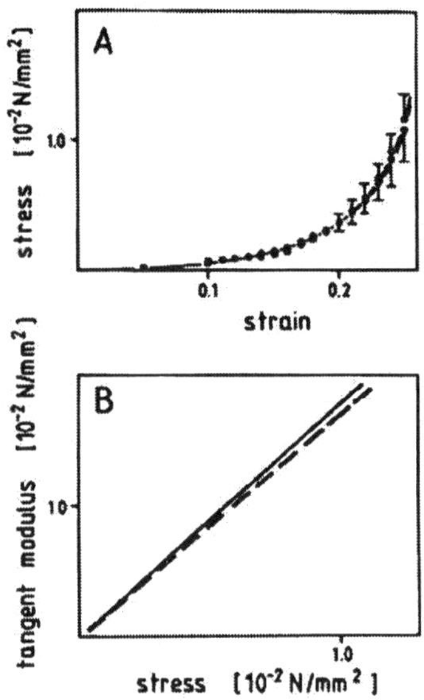

Figure 3: Stress-strain relationship ***(A)*** *and tangent modulus-stress relationship* ***(B)*** *in normal (---) and thyrotoxic, hypertrophied rat myocardium (—). According to [7].*
Please note that there is no difference in myocardial diastolic compliance.

In contrast, in the Goldblatt model (eight weeks of renal artery constriction) and in the spontaneously hypertensive rat, we found increased stiffness which was associated with a significant increase in interstitial space (morphometric data) and in collagen content (hydroxyproline determination) in both cases (Figure 4 and 5) [7,8].

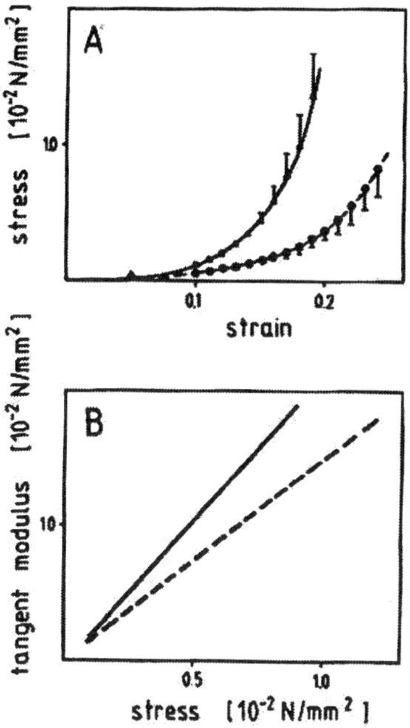

*Figure 4: Stress-strain relationship **(A)** and tangent modulus-stress relationship **(B)** in normal (---) and Goldblatt hypertrophied rat myocardium (—; one clip; two kidneys; 8 weeks). According to [7,8].*
Please note that diastolic compliance dramatically decreased within 8 weeks of arterial hypertension.

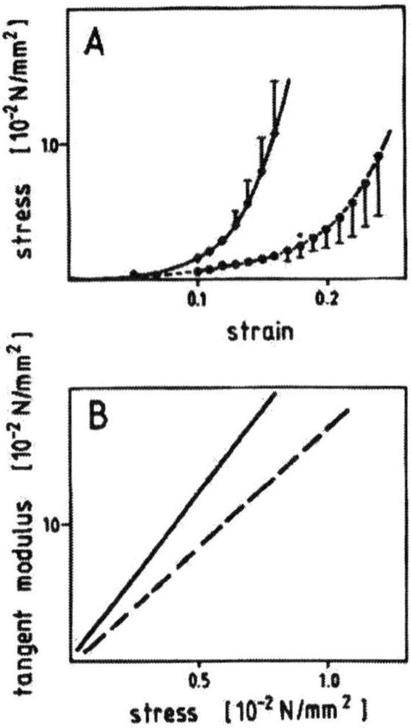

*Figure 5: Stress-strain relationship (**A**) and tangent modulus-stress relationship (**B**) in normal (---) and pressure overload rat myocardium (—; SHR spontaneously hypertensive rats; 80 weeks old). According to [7,8].*
Please note that diastolic compliance dramatically increased due to arterial hypertension.

8.3.2. Stress-Strain Relationships Derived from Whole Heart Experiments from Animals

Our group was able to demonstrate increased stiffness for Goldblatt myocardium by calculating myocardial stiffness from pressure-volume relations and wall thickness [9,10]. More importantly, Brilla et al. reported on increases in the slope of tangent elastic moduluIs versus stress function in SHR rats which were reversible by long-term treatment with the angiotensin-converting-enzyme inhibitor lisinopril (Figure 6) [11].

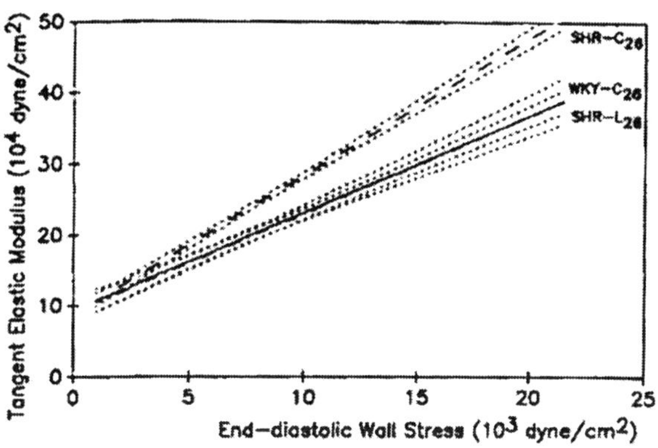

Figure 6: Tangent elastic modulus as a function of enddiastolic wall stress: Compliance is decreased in SHR rats compared to WKY rats. Treatment with lisinopril (angiotensin-converting-enzyme inhibitor) reverses the myocardial stiffness increase to normal. According to [11].

8.3.3. Stress-Strain Relationship in Isolated Human Muscle Strip Preparations

To our knowledge, complete resting length-tension relations have not been published systemically for human cardiac tissues. However, there is no doubt that failing human myocardium shows steeper resting length-tension curves than non-failing (see Figure 7).

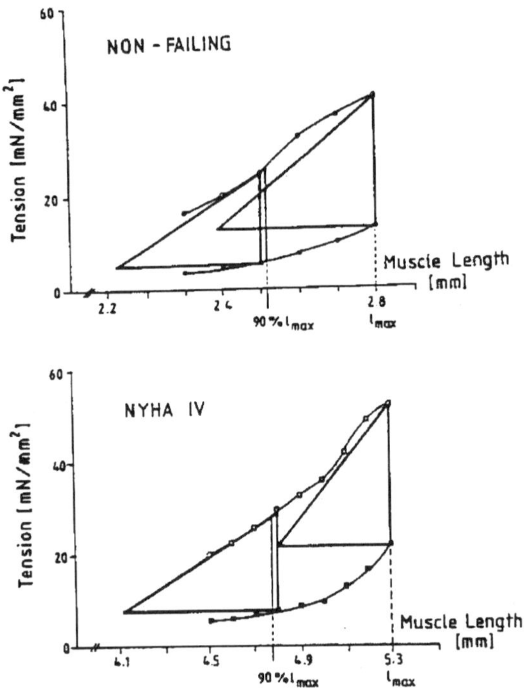

Figure 7: Length-tension curves in normal and endstage failing human left ventricular muscle preparations. Note that the resting tension curve is steeper in failing than in nonfailing myocardium. Resting tension at optimum length l_{max} is also higher in failing than in nonfailing human myocardium.
According to [12].

We found resting tension at l_{max} to be significantly higher in failing than in non-failing human myocardium (Figure 8) [12,13].

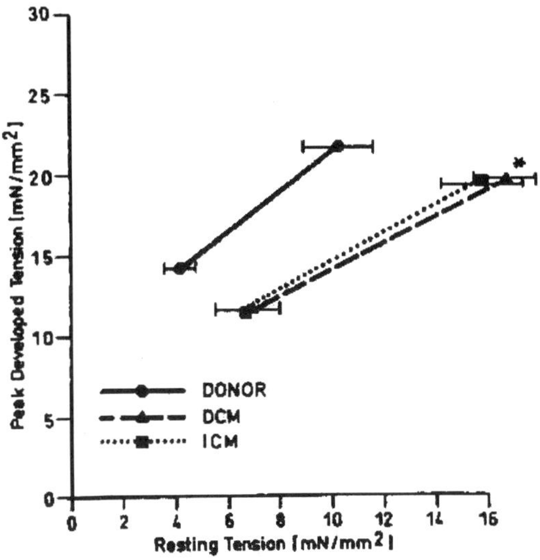

Figure 8: Peak developed tension as a function of resting tension in normal human myocardium (DONOR) and failing human myocardium (DCM, dilated cardiomyopathy; ICM, ischemic cardiomyopathy). Whereas peak developed force is not different between groups when measured at optimum length, resting tension is much higher in failing than in nonfailing left ventricular myocardium. According to [13].

8.3.4. Stress-Strain Relationships Derived from the Human Heart in Vivo

In an excellent invasive study, Hess et al. [14] were able to completely analyze the passive elastic properties of left ventricular myocardium in patients with aortic stenosis – before and after aortic valve replacement. These authors did not only show that myocardial stiffness is increased in patients with left ventricular hypertrophy, they also demonstrated the association to interstitial fibrosis, i.e., collagen formation, and the principal reversibility of that process after valve replacement and regression of cardiac hypertrophy [14].

8.3.5. Impaired Relaxation in Human Failing Cardiac Muscle

A number of studies using isolated human cardiac muscle have shown relevant impaired relaxation which resulted obviously in an increase in diastolic tone, when high stimulation rate was applied [15,16]. The most recent and interesting study was completed by Hasenfuss et al. [17]. These authors found diastolic failure at high stimulation rates in about half of the preparations whereas diastolic tone was not altered by high stimulation rate in the other half of preparations. These observations were associated with molecular changes regarding the calcium-sodium-exchanger on the one hand and the sarcoplasmic calcium ATPase on the other (Figure 9).

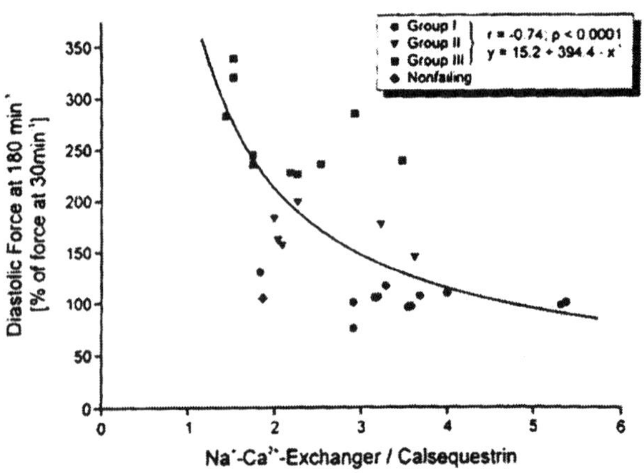

Figure 9: Relation between diastolic force (contracture) and sodium-calcium exchanger in failing human ventricular muscle preparations. The lower the sodium-calcium exchanger concentration, the higher diastolic force, i.e., contracture tension. According to [17].

These data provoke a very interesting hypothesis for diastolic heart failure and may open differential therapeutic strategies for patients. However, in the human being in vivo, we did not find this type of diastolic failure when applying heart rates as high as 140 bpm in patients with dilated cardiomyopathy: Increases in heart rate did not enhance left ventricular enddiastolic pressure despite unchanged enddiastolic volumes (see Table 1) [18].

	Normal ventricles (n=8)			**Dilated ventricles (n=9)**		
	LVEPD [mmHg]	LVEDV [ml]	dP/dt_{max} [mmHg/sec]	LVEPD [mmHg]	LVEDV [ml]	dP/dt_{max} [mmHg/sec]
P_1	13	130	1388	15	288	855
100/min	16	120	1526**	13	287	879
120/min	13	n.d.	1658**	15	n.d.	889
140/min	14	110*	1671**	17	285	920

*Table 1: Influence of heart rate (stimulation rate) on left ventricular enddiastolic pressure (LVEDP), on left ventricular enddiastolic volume (LVEDV), and maximum pressure/rise (dP/dt_{max}) in patients with normal and dilated ventricles. P_1, lowest pacing rate (~ 85/min). * $p<0.05$; ** $p<0.01$. Note that LVEDP and LVEDV are unchanged in dilated ventricles with increasing stimulation rates. According to [18].*

8.4. Discussion

8.4.1. Interstitial Fibrosis

From a molecular point of view, the most extensive work on interstitial fibrosis has been performed by Brilla and Weber [19,20]. They could demonstrate that (1) the renin-angiotensin-system is involved as well as (2) aldosterone (Table 2).

	HTN	LVH	LV/RV-FIB
RHT	+	+	+
AL	+	+	+
RHT+S	+	+	-
AL+S	+	+	-
AL+SS	-	-	-

Table 2: Prevention of myocardial fibrosis by application of spironolacton. HTN, hypertension; LVH, left ventricular LV/RV-FIB, fibrosis of the left and right ventricle; RHT, renal hypertension; AL, hyperaldesteronism; S, treatment with spironolacton (low dose); SS, treatment with spironolacton (high dose). According to [20].

However, in both instances, spironolactone administration, an aldosterone antagonist, was able to prevent interstitial fibrosis (see Table 2). These observations – in conjunction with the previously mentioned study [11] showing reversibility of interstitial fibrosis and myocardial stiffness due to ACE inhibition in spontaneously hypertension rats – underline the importance of the renin-angiotensin-system in diastolic dysfunction.

8.4.2. Impaired Relaxation

For a long time, impaired left ventricular relaxation has been described and discussed as a possible mechanism which may come into play in diastolic heart failure in addition to structural changes of the myocardium due to fibrosis. Furthermore, permanent or transient ischemia may lead to disturbances of diastolic compliance due to myocardial contracture and reversible formations of rigor bonds between actin and myosin [21].

However, a very attractive hypothesis has been proposed by Hasenfuss et al. [17]: Disturbances of calcium homeostasis may lead to an increased diastolic tone when the myocardium is stressed to higher heart rates. These functional diastolic disturbances may be related to differential expression of the Ca^{2+}-ATPase and the calcium-sodium-exchanger. However, at the moment, we have no clear data at hand that these observations may play a role in the clinical situation.

REFERENCES

1) Mirsky I: Elastic properties of the myocardium: A quantitative approach with physiological and clinical application. In: Berne RM (ed). Handbook of Physiology. The Cardiovascular System. Washington, DC, American Physiological Society 1979, pp 497-531

2) Hepp A, Hansis M, Gülch R, Jacob R: Left ventricular isovolumic pressure-volume relations, "diastolic tone" and contractility in the rat heart after physiological training. Basic Res Cardiol 1974;69:516-532

3) Spann JF, Covell JW, Eckberg KL, Sonnenblick EH, Ross J, Braunwald E: Contractile performance of the hypertrophied and chronically failing cat ventricle. Am J Physiol 1972;223:1150-1157

4) Buccino RA, Harris E, Spann JF, Sonnenblick EH: Response of myocardial connective tissue to development of experimental hypertrophy. Am J Physiol 1969;216:425-428

5) Bing OHL, Matsushita S, Fanburg BL, Levine HJ: Mechanical properties of rat cardiac muscle during experimental hypertrophy. Circ Res 1971;28:234-245

6) Alpert NR, Hamrell BB, Holpen W: Mechanical and biochemical correlates of cardiac hypertrophy. Circ Res 1974;34&35:71-82

7) Holubarsch Ch, Holubarsch Th, Jacob R, Medugorac I, Thiedemann K-U: Passive elastic properties of myocardium in different models and stages of hypertrophy: A study comparing mechanical, chemical, and morphometric parameters. In: Perspectives in Cardiovascular Research, 7, Myocardial Hypertrophy and Failure. Alpert NR. Raven Press. New York 1983;323-336

8) Thiedemann K-U, Holubarsch Ch, Medugorac I, Jacob R: Myocardial stiffness and connective tissue content in pressure induced cardiac hypertrophy. Basic Res Cardiol 1983;78:140-155

9) Jacob R, Kissling G: Left ventricular dynamics and myocardial function in Goldblatt hypertension of the rat. Biochemical, morphological and electrophysiological correlates. In: The Heart in Hypertension. Strauer BE (ed). Springer. Berlin, Heidelberg, New York 1981;89-106

10) Vogt M, Jacob R, Noma K, Onegi B, Rupp H: Chronic cardiac reactions. III. Factors involved in the development of structural dilatation. In: Cardiac Energetics. Jacob R, Just H, Holubarsch Ch (eds). Steinkopff Verlag Darmstadt. Springer Verlag New York. Basic Res Cardiol 1987;82 (Suppl II): 161-172

11) Brilla ChG, Janicki JS, Weber KT: Cardiac reparative effects of lisinopril in rats with genetic hypertension and left ventricular hypertrophy. Circulation 1991;83:1771-1779

12) Holubarsch Ch, Lüdemann J, Wiessner S, Ruf Th, Schulte-Baukloh H, Schmidt-Schweda S, Pieske B, Posival H, Just H: Shortening versus isometric contractions in isolated human failing and non-failing left ventricular myocardium. Dependency of external work and force on muscle length, heart rate and inotropic stimulation. Cardiovascular Research 1998;37:46-57

13) Holubarsch Ch, Ruf Th, Goldstein DJ, Ashton RC, Nickl W, Pieske B, Pioch K, Lüdemann J, Wiesner S, Hasenfuss G, Posival H, Just H, Burkhoff D: Existence of the Frank-Starling mechanism in the failing human heart. Circulation 1996;94:683-689

14) Hess OM, Schneider J, Koch R, Bauert C, Grimm J, Krayenbuehl HP: Diastolic function and myocardial hypertrophy. Special reference to normalized viscoelastic data. Circulation 1981;63:360-371

15) Gwathmey IK, Slawsky MT, Hajjar RJ, Briggs CM, Morgan JP: Role of intracellular calcium handling in force-interval relationships of human ventricular myocardium. J Clin Invest 1990;85:1599-1613

16) Barry WH, Bridge JHB: Intracellular calcium homeostasis in cardiac myocytes. Circulation 1993;87:1806-1815

17) Hasenfuss G, Schillinger W, Lehnart SE, Preuss M, Pieske B, Maier LS, Prestle J, Minami K, Just H: Relationship between Na^{+}-Ca^{2+}-exchanger protein levels and diastolic dysfunction in failing human myocardium. Circulation 1999;99:641-648

18) Hasenfuss G, Holubarsch Ch, Hermann HP, Astheimer K, Pieske B, Just H: Influence of the force-frequency relationship on haemodynamics and left ventricular function in patients with non-failing hearts and in patients with dilated cardiomyopathy. European Heart J 1994;15:164-170

19) Brilla CG, Pick R, Tau LB, Janicki JS, Weber KT: Remodeling of the rat right and left ventricle in experimental hypertension. Circ Res 1990;67:1355-1364

20) Weber KT, Brilla CG: Pathologic hypertrophy and the cardiac interstitium: Fibrosis and the renin-angiotensin-aldosterone system. Circulation 1991;83:1849-1865

21) Holubarsch Ch, Alpert NR, Goulette R, Mulieri LA: Heat production during hypoxic contracture of rat myocardium. Circ Res 1982;51:777-786

9. THE E_{MAX} AND THE PVA CONCEPT

9.1. Introduction

In search for a ventricular index of left ventricular contractility which should be independent of preload and afterload as much as possible (see also Chapter III), Suga and Sugawa in 1974 [1] developed the E_{max} concept (end-systolic pressure-volume ratio) which was based on the time-varying elastance theory of ventricular contraction. This theory can be best described by a spring as demonstrated in Figure 1: at end-diastole (Figure 1A), the thin spring symbolizes the compliant chamber wall, i.e., elastance is low. At end-systole, the thick spring symbolizes the stiffened chamber wall, i.e., elastance has increased and has become maximum (Figure 1B).

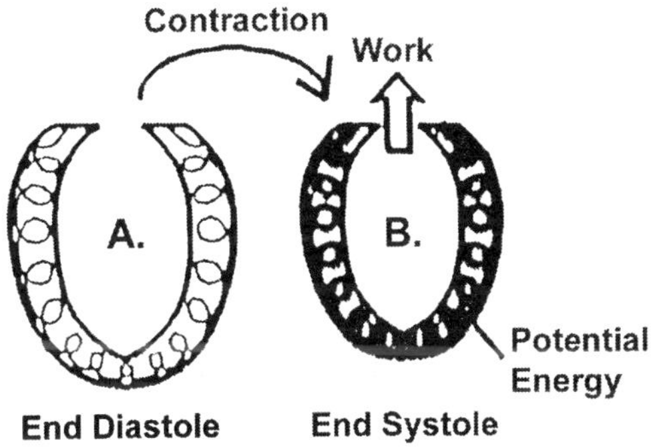

*Figure 1: **A.** The left ventricle at end-diastole represented by a thin spring, i.e., low elastance. **B.** The left ventricle at end-systole represented by a thick spring, i.e., maximum elastance. During contraction, work has been performed and potential energy is stored in the spring. According to [7].*

When plotting time-varying elastance ($E_{(t)}$) as a function of volume, a family of linear relations is obtained each indicating the instantaneous elastance at a certain point of time for contractions starting from different filling volumes. The steepest relation, i.e., the maximum elastance is called E_{max} (see Figure 2A).

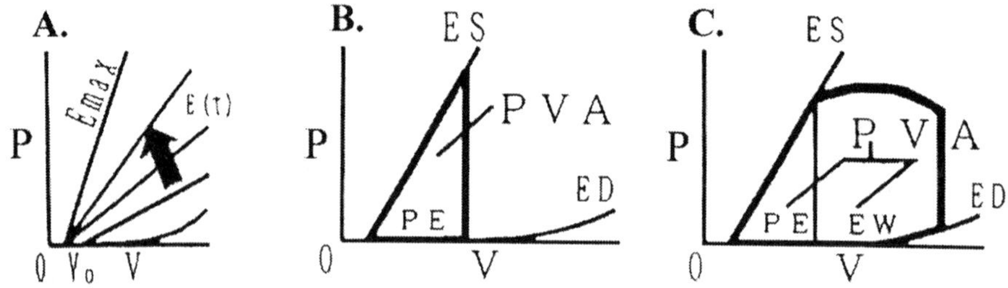

Figure 2: ***A.*** *Counterclockwise rotation of the instantaneous P-V line during systole.* ***B.*** *Isovolumic contraction without external work output but increment in potential energy.* ***C.*** *Ejecting contraction with external work output and increase in potential energy. P, pressure; V, volume; PVA, pressure-volume area; PE, potential energy; EW, external work; ES, end-systole; ED, end-diastole. According to [7].*

Because the increment in elastance is energetically represented by both an increase in potential energy stored in the time-varying elastic wall and the generation of external work (pressure-volume work), the time-varying elastance approach can be changed to the pressure-volume-area-(PVA-)concept [2]. Figure 2B explains this concept for an isovolumic contraction and Figure 2C for a blood ejecting contraction (isotonic).

In case of an isovolumic contraction, the energy involved is all potential energy as described by a single term, i.e., the area between the E_{max} line, the abscissa (volume) and the isovolumic vertical pressure line (equals PVA, Figure 2B). In case of an isotonic (afterloaded or working) contraction, PVA is composed of external work (pressure-volume work) plus potential energy as given by the small area between the E_{max} line, the abscissa (volume), and the vertical pressure line during relaxation (Figure 2C). In an isovolumic contraction, all the potential energy is released in form of heat, whereas in an ejecting contraction the energy is released in form of both mechanical energy (external work) and heat.

This concept has been developed and proven for a variety of conditions by using an isolated but cross-circulated dog heart (see below in Methods).

In such an experimental setting, it was no experimental problem to measure oxygen consumption of the left ventricular myocardium (MVO_2) and to correlate MVO_2 to the pressure-volume area. As a result, a linear relationship was obtained (Figure 3) with a slope a, which gives oxygen cost of PVA. The reciprocal value of a (1/a) is the contractile efficiency.

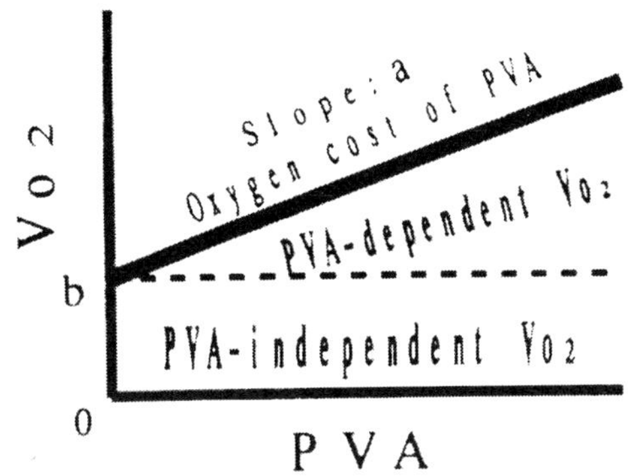

Figure 3: Oxygen consumption of the left ventricle (VO_2) as a function of pressure-volume area (PVA). Slope a indicates oxygen cost of PVA, and intercept b represents PVA-independent VO_2 (see text). According to [7].

The linear relationship between MVO_2 and PVA also shows a relevant intercept b, which is significantly different from zero. This intercept b represents the MVO_2 which is independent of generation of PVA and is certainly composed of oxygen consumption due to resting metabolism on the one hand and oxygen consumption involved in calcium handling on the other (see Results of this chapter, but also Chapter 4).

9.2. Methods

The contractility index E_{max} as well as the PVA concept have been developed in the isolated cross-circulated dog heart [3, 4, 5]. The main reason for the excision and isolation of the heart is the need to control perfectly preload and afterload as well as to perform exact measurements of volume and pressure. On the other hand, physiological coronary blood flow has to be provided which must be independent on the pressure developed and the work generated by the isolated heart. To guarantee physiological coronary blood flow independent on contractile performance and loading conditions of the heart under study, Suga and Sugawa developed the experimental model of the cross-circulated dog heart.

9.2.1. The heart preparation

For this purpose, two mongrel dogs are needed: one for providing coronary circulation, from the other the heart is used for the study. In this model of cross-circulation, the ascending aorta of the heart under study is connected by the left subclavian artery, and some connecting tubes to the common carotid arteries of the supporting dog, whereas the right ventricle is connected to the jugular vein of the supporting dog for venous reflow. From the opened left atrium a thin rubber balloon is placed into the left ventricle. This balloon is connected to a volume servo pump so that the volume of the balloon and thereby the left ventricular volume is controlled.

The arterial blood pressure of the support dog provides the coronary perfusion pressure of the heart preparation, which was constant at about 90 mmHg and absolutely independent on the pressures and volumes within the heart preparation. Heart rate was controlled by means of electrical stimulation via a pair of electrodes. For on-line measurements of left ventricular pressure, a miniature pressure gauge was placed inside the apical end of the rubber balloon.

An ECG was detected from the epicardium and used for electrical trigger of the volume servo pump [3,4,5].

9.2.2. Oxygen Consumption Measurements

Total coronary blood flow was measured by means of an electromagnetic flowmeter placed in the middle of a coronary venous tubing that drained all venous coronary blood to the right heart [6].

The right ventricle was maintained at zero volume to keep oxygen consumption of the right ventricle as low as possible.

By means of the oxyhemoglobin percent saturation of the coronary arterial and venous blood the coronary arteriovenous oxygen content difference was determined. This parameter was multiplied by measured total coronary blood flow and divided by heart rate yielding MVO_2/beat [6].

9.3. Results

9.3.1. The E_{max} and the PVA Concept in the Isolated Dog Heart

In the experimental isolated and instrumented dog heart one can obtain the E_{max} line by varying the following parameters: The preload or end-diastolic filling volume (see Figure 4A), the afterload (see Figure 4B), and both of these (see Figure 4C).

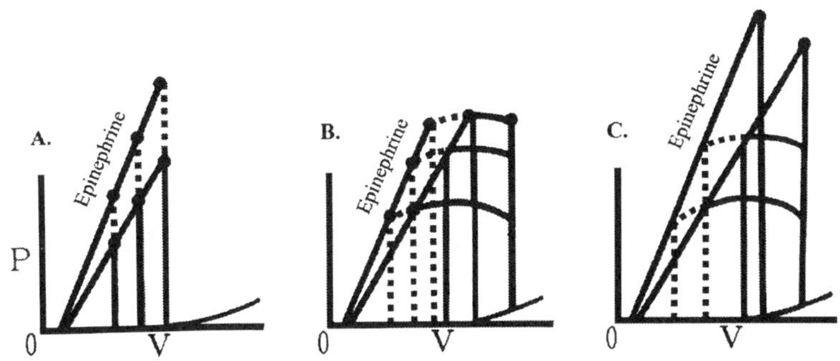

*Figure 4: **A.** Pressure-volume relations obtained by isovolumic contractions: control and epinephrine. **B.** Pressure-volume relations obtained by afterloaded ejecting contractions: control and epinephrine. C. Pressure-volume relations obtained by isovolumic and afterloaded ejecting contractions: control and epinephrine.*

Because all of the contractions in Figure 4 A, B, and C end at end-systole on the linear E_{max} line, the slope of it is greatly independent on preload and afterload [3,4].

When correlating the PVA area, i.e., pressure-volume work plus potential energy, to the corresponding myocardial oxygen consumption, a linear relationship is obtained with a slope a representing PVA-dependent oxygen consumption and an intercept b representing PVA-independent oxygen consumption (Figure 5A). Each increase in E_{max} is supposed to either increase the intercept b (parallel upward shift of the MVO_2 vs. PVA relation (Figure 5A)) or to alter the slope a (steeper MVO_2 vs. PVA relation (Figur 5B)) [7].

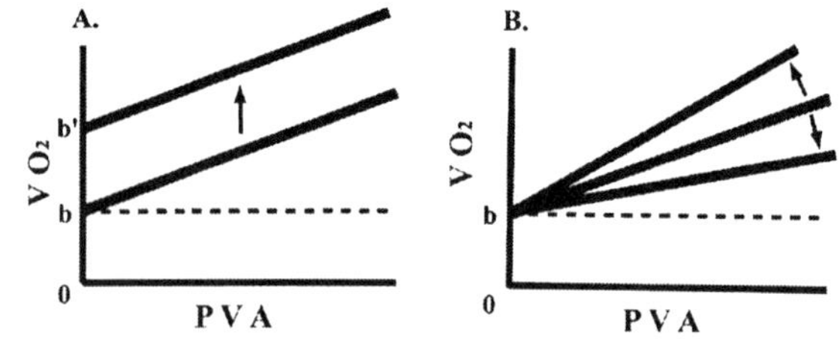

*Figure 5: **A.** Positive inotropic compounds like epinephrine, calcium, phosphodiesterase inhibitors, digitalis and others, all shift the VO_2 vs PVA relation upwards in a parallel manner (increase in intercept b) indicating an increase in calcium turnover. **B**. Potential changes in myocardial efficiency on the level of contractile proteins are demonstrated: However, positive inotropes do not increase the slope of the relation. Stunning and acidosis decrease the slope thereby increasing myocardial efficiency at the level of contractile proteins.*

9.3.2. Acute Changes in E_{max}

All positive inotropic interventions tested so far (catecholamines, calcium, digitalis, paired pulse stimulation, as well as phosphodiesterase inhibitors) increase E_{max} as shown in Figure 4A-C [7]. Despite this increase in E_{max}, the slope of the MVO_2 vs. PVA relation, i.e., the oxygen cost of PVA is unaltered (Figure 5A) [6,7]. The only change of the MVO_2 vs PVA relation is the increase in the intercept b (Figure 5A) indicating PVA-independent mechanisms like resting metabolism or calcium handling. The only two acute interventions that have been shown to alter the oxygen cost of PVA is stunning and acidosis [8, 9]. However, these two pathophysiological states are characterized by a decrease in the slope of MVO_2 vs. PVA function, i.e., going along with enhanced contractile efficiency (Figure 5B).

9.3.3. Chronic changes of Oxygen cost of PVA

The question of whether chronic diseases like hypothyroidism, thyrotoxicosis, and cardiac hypertrophy may alter the MVO_2 cost of PVA is answered controversially: Whereas a decreased efficiency, i.e., greater MVO_2 cost of PVA has been found for the thyrotoxic rabbit heart [10], contractile efficiency was unaltered in hypertrophied canine heart as compared to euthyroid hearts [11]. For hypertrophied and failing canine hearts, only preliminary reports have been published which are even more conflicting: one group [12] reports an unchanged contractile efficiency in failing canine myocardium, whereas the other [13] finds a decrease in oxygen costs of PVA for the failing canine hearts. This data is especially conflicting, because both groups used the same canine model of pacing-induced cardiomyopathy.

9.4. Discussion

The development of cardiovascular research in the past has been greatly influenced by the E_{max} and the PVA concept. E_{max} as a load-independent term was used to describe left ventricular dynamics and alterations of the inotropic state. Using the same theory for the evaluation of left ventricular energetics, i.e., creating the MVO_2-PVA relation, allowed the separation between load-independent mechanisms, i.e., calcium handling, and resting metabolism, and mechanical energy liberation as described by PVA, i.e., cross-bridge dynamics (see also Chapter IV).

However, scientists have identified a number of shortcomings of the time-varying elastance theory. Limitations include (1) some fundamental assumptions, (2) the phenomenological description of the left ventricular dynamics rather than an analysis of molecular processes of cardiac muscle, and (3) the sensitivity of the MVO_2-PVA relation for detection of fundamental molecular alterations which take place due to acute and chronic interventions.

Ad (1): The E_{max}-concept is based on the assumption that all contractions of the ventricle end on a linear line (E_{max}) at end-systole independent on preload (diastolic filling) and afterload. However, it has been demonstrated that this assumption is a simplification of the physiology of the heart: Burkhoff et al. [14] have demonstrated that E_{max} lines constructed from isovolumetric contraction are different from those obtained from ejecting beats.

The same authors demonstrated that the E_{max} line is non-linear and, furthermore, the degree of non-linearity depends on the inotropic state [15].

Ad (2): Regarding molecular processes involved in cardiac contraction, the E_{max} and the PVA concept have brought about important views inside the cardiac muscle, especially the separation between PVA independent and PVA dependent energetic processes. However, it may be that alterations of cross-bridge cycling mechanisms are not well detected with this methodological approach especially when compared to other methods (see chapters IV, V, VI).

Ad (3): In the dog heart using the PVA concept no changes in mechanical efficiency have been found for acute (catecholamines) [6,7] and chronic interventions (hyperthyroidism and pacing-induced cardiomyopathy) [11,12]. This negative result may be explained by the low sensitivity of the method. Using either isometric contraction economy parameters (see Chapter IV) or the frequency response method (see Chapter VI), alterations of cross-bridge cycling rates have been found. And indeed, when Suga et al. [16] theoretically analyzed the relationship between isometric economy and maximum mechanical efficiency based on Hill's equation and published skeletal muscle data, they found that an increase in isometric economy by a factor of 100 would only double maximum mechanical efficiency, or a twofold decrease in isometric economy would reduce maximum mechanical efficiency of the contractile proteins, for example, from 0.55 to 0.50. Therefore, a biological relevant change in cross-bridge cycling mechanisms may result in an only small change in mechanical efficiency, which may hardly be detectable [6, 7]. However, even a small change in mechanical efficiency may be of great biological significance - in the long term run. This insensitivity of the PVA-MVO_2 relation may also explain why mechanical efficiency changes are detectable in the hyperthyroid rabbit but no in the hyperthyroid canine heart, and explain the conflicting data of the pacing-induced cardiomyopathy model of the dog heart.

REFERENCES

1) Suga H, Sagawa K: Instantaneous pressure-volume relationships and their ratio in the excised supported canine left ventricle. Circ Res 1974;35:117-126

2) Suga H: Ventricular energetics. Physiol Rev 1990;70:217-277

3) Suga H, Sagawa K, Shonkas AA: Load independence of the instantaneous pressure-volume ratio of the canine left ventricle and effects of epinephrine and heart rate on the ratio. Circ Res 1973;32:314-322

4) Suga H, Sagawa K: Instantaneous pressure-volume relationships and their ratio in the excised, supported canine left ventricle. Circ Res 1974;35:117-126

5) Suga H, Hayashi T, Shirahata M: Ventricular systolic pressure volume area as predictor of cardiac oxygen consumption. Am J Physiol 1981;240:H39-44

6) Suga H, Hisano R, Goto Y, Yamada O, Igarashi Y: Effect of positive inotropic agents on the relation between oxygen consumption and systolic pressure-volume area in canine left ventricles. Circ Res 1983;53:306-318

7) Suga H, Takaki M, Matsubara H, Goto Y: Energy costs of PVA and E_{max}: Constancy and Variability. In: Cardiac Energetics: From E_{max} to pressure-volume area. Eds.: LeWinter MM, Suga H, Watkins WM. Kluwer Academic Publishers 1995, pp 1-15

8) Ohgoshi Y, Goto Y, Futaki S, Yaku H, Kawaguchi O, Suga H: Increased oxygen cost of contractility in stunned myocardium of dog. Circ Res 1991;69:975-988

9) Hata K, Goto Y, Kawagushi O, Takasago T, Saeki A, Nishioka T, Suga H: Hypercapnic acidosis increases oxygen cost of contractility in the dog left ventricle. Am J Physiol 1994;266:H730-H740

10) Goto Y, Slinker BK, LeWinter MM: Decreased contractile efficiency and increased nonmechanical energy cost in hyperthyroid rabbit heart: relation between O_2 consumption and systolic pressure-volume area or force-time integral. Circ Res 1990;66:999-1011

11) Suga H, Tanaka N, Ohgoshi Y, Saeki Y, Nakanishi T, Futaki S, Yaku H, Goto Y: Hyperthyroid dog left ventricle has the same oxygen consumption versus pressure-volume area (PVA) relation as euthyroid dog. Heart Vessels 1991;6:71-83

12) Goto Y, Yaku H, Ohgoshi Y, Futaki S, Kawaguchi O, Hata K, Takasago T, Saeki A, Suga H: Left ventricular mechanics and energetics in dogs with pacing-induced heart failure. Circulation 1991;84 (Suppl II):0379

13) Wolff MR, DeTombe PP, Harasawa Y, Burkhoff D, Hunter WC, Gerstenblith G, Kass DA: Energetics of the failing heart: Greater chemomechanical efficiency but increased inotropic cost. Circulation 1991;84 (Suppl II):0378

14) Burkhoff D et al: Contractile strength and mechanical efficiency of left ventricle are enhanced by physiological overload. Am J Physiol 1991;60:H569-H578

15) Burkhoff et al: Contractility-dependent curvilinearity of end-systolic pressure-volume relations. Am J Physiol 1987;21:H1218-H1227

17) Suga H, Goto Y, Hata K, et al: Constant efficiency versus variable economy of cardiac contraction. Jpn Heart J 1992;33:213-227

10. OXYGEN CONSUMPTION MEASUREMENTS OF THE MYOCARDIUM IN THE HUMAN BEING

10.1. Introduction

One might argue that the best way to study myocardial energetics is to measure the myocardial oxygen consumption of patients and healthy subjects in vivo – possibly before and after an acute or chronic pharmacological intervention. Although this idea is intriguing, there is a number of limitations for such a procedure. (1) Such a kind of procedure is invasive and time-consuming, and therefore some ethical considerations come into play (see below). (2) In the whole organism, any inotropic or vasodilating pharmacological intervention is necessarily followed by reflex neuroendocrine mechanisms which make interpretations of altered myocardial oxygen consumption invalid or at least complicated. In order to overcome this problem, myocardial oxygen consumption must be considered in relation to the respective hemodynamic variables, i.e., stress-time integral, peak systolic stress, pressure-volume area, contraction velocity and others (see below). (3) Measurements of myocardial oxygen consumption – in contrast to hemodynamic measurements – need long periods of steady state conditions.

It was the merit of Richard Bing [1] to conduct the first measurements of myocardial oxygen consumption in men in 1949 using N_2O which served as a tracer for myocardial perfusion analysis. Interestingly, he found efficiency, i.e., the quotient of pressure-volume work divided by myocardial oxygen consumption, of about 25 % for normal hearts (see below).

10.2. Methods

10.2.1. Measurements of Myocardial Oxygen Consumption

In order to measure myocardial blood perfusion of the whole heart, it is not sufficient to analyze regional blood flow in one coronary artery as can be performed very accurately by a Doppler-tipped guidewire [2,3]. Rather a method is needed by which global myocardial perfusion of the whole heart (left ventricle) is obtained. In principle, this can be achieved by two different methods: (1) An inert gas (N_2O or argon) is applied the concentration of which is measured simultaneously in the aorta and in the sinus coronarius allowing recalculation of global myocardial perfusion [1]. (2) Another method, which was not used in our hands, is the coronary sinus thermodilution method [4,5].

In the past, we have successfully performed investigations in about 300 patients to study myocardial oxygen consumption.

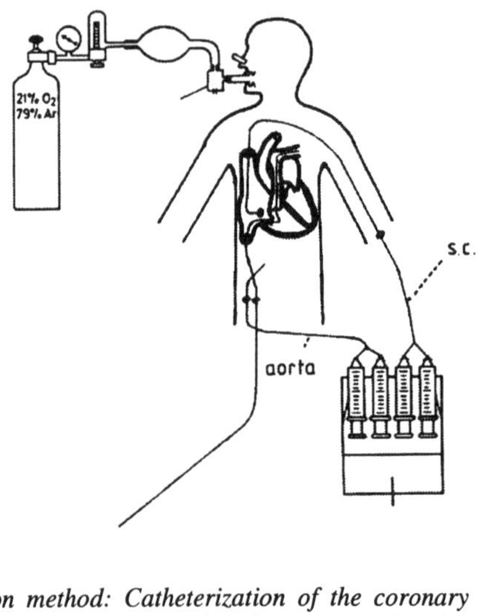

Figure 1: The argon method: Catheterization of the coronary sinus (S.C.) was accomplished through the left brachial vein. A pigtail catheter is positioned in the aorta via the right femoral artery. During a period of 5 min during which the patient is breathing 79% argon/21% oxygen, blood samples are continuously withdrawn from the aorta and the sinus coronarius.

As shown in Figure 1, a pigtail catheter is placed in the aorta via the femoral artery approach, a multipurpose catheter is positioned in the sinus coronarius via the left cubital vein approach, so that blood can be withdrawn simultaneously by a special suction pump.

Over a period of five minutes, the patient is breathing a mixture of 21 % oxygen and 79 % argon. Argon saturation curves are shown in Figure 2.

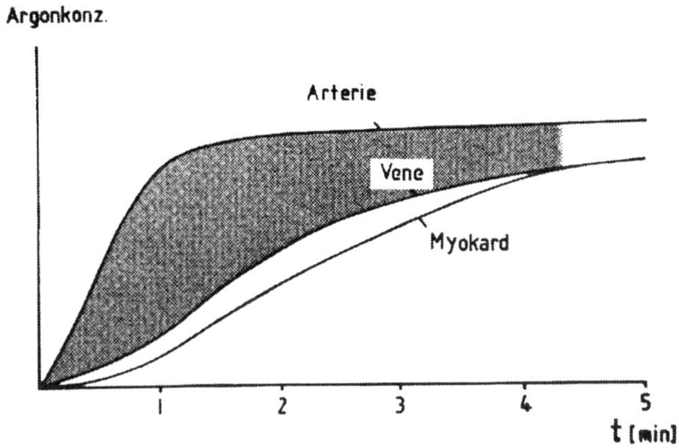

Figure 2: The argon method: Argon concentrations in the aorta and sinus coronarius as a function of time. The area between these two sigmoidal concentration curves is inversely related to myocardial blood flow which can be calculated according to Kety and Smith [6].

The area between the arterial (left) and coronary sinus (venous, right) sigmoid curves reflects myocardial blood flow in a reciprocal relationship. According to the Kety and Schmidt formula [6], the myocardial blood flow can be calculated from the respective argon blood concentrations as measured by gas chromatography [7,8,9]. In order to evaluate myocardial oxygen consumption, it was also necessary to define the arterial-coronary-sinus-oxygen-content-difference (ml/100 ml). This can be accomplished by oxygen saturation measurements using oximetry (AO Unistat Oximeter, Munich, Germany). Myocardial oxygen consumption can then be calculated by multiplying myocardial blood flow times the arterial-coronary-sinus-oxygen-content-difference. Myocardial oxygen consumption per beat (µl/beat/100 g muscle tissue) is easily obtained from myocardial oxygen consumption per minute and heart rate.

10.2.2. Determination of Mechanical Parameters

As outlined before, interpretations of myocardial oxygen consumption are only possible, when hemodynamic variables are measured and taken into account. In order to evaluate these hemodynamic and mechanical parameters, left ventricular pressure was measured by means of a Millar microtipped catheter pressure transducer (PC-485, 87) during ventriculography. The latter was performed at 50 frames/sec by power injection of 40ml nonionic contrast solution. From each cine frame, left ventricular volume and wall thickness was analyzed by the Sandler-Dodge method [10,11,12]. Then, for each instantaneous volume, the corresponding pressure volume can be attributed (Figure 3A and 3B).

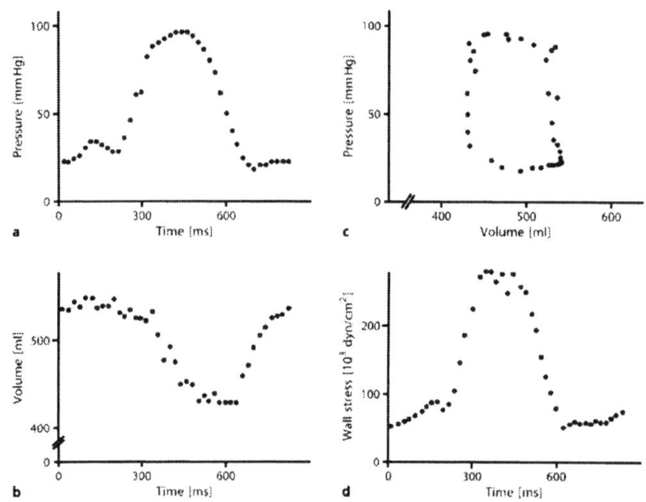

*Figure 3: Pressure, volume, and left ventricular wall stress as analyzed from a patient with dilated cardiomyopathy: **a)** Pressure as a function of time (measured by Millar-tip pressure transducer). **b)** Volume as a function of time (analyzed from angiographic cine frames). **c)** Pressure as a function of volume (constructed from diagrams a) and b)). **d)** Systolic wall stress as calculated according to [12].*

For a long time, one has recognized that geometrical factors of the left ventricle play a decisive role regarding myocardial mechanics and energetics. This fact was first described by Laplace (Figure 4A) assuming a thin-walled sphere [13]. Mirsky in 1979 [14] further developed this concept to a thick-walled ellipsoid (Figure 4B).

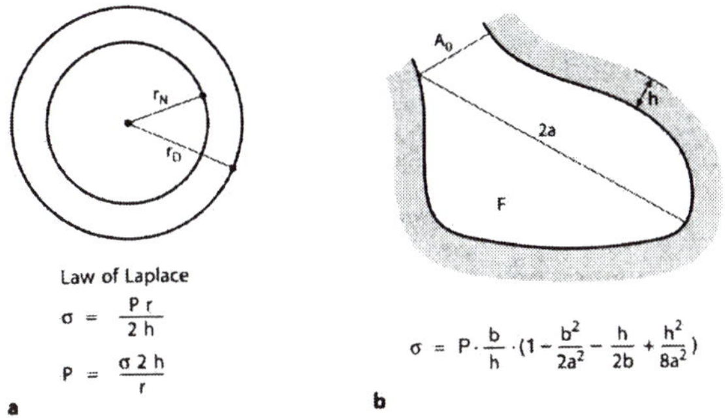

*Figure 4: Formulas of Laplace and Mirsky: Using the equation of La Place, left ventricular chamber is assumed to be a thin-walled sphere (**a**); using the equation of Mirsky, left ventricular chamber is assumed to be a thick-walled ellipsoid (**b**).*

The parameters which can be derived from the above mentioned concepts and which are thought to determine myocardial oxygen consumption are the following:

(1) Peak systolic wall stress (Figure 3D).
(2) The pressure-volume work (Figure 3C).
(3) The stress-time integral (Figure 3D).
(4) dP/dt_{max} (maximum rate of pressure rize).
(5) Mean velocity of circumferential fiber shortening.

Ad (1): Myocardial wall stress is calculated from pressure and geometrical data according to the formula

$$S = P \times b/h \times (1 - b^2/2a^2 - h/2b + h^2/8a^2)$$

under the assumption of a thick-walled ellipsoid according to Mirsky [14] and v. Herrath et al. [12], when S equals stress, P equals pressure, and h is wall thickness, a is major hemiaxis, and b is minor hemiaxis.

Ad (2): Pressure-volume work is simply the area of the pressure-volume loop shown in Figure 3C.

Ad (3): The stress-time integral is obtained from calculated stress values obtained over time, i.e., every 20 msec, for a whole heart cycle (see Figure 3D).

Ad (4): dP/dt_{max} is directly obtained by electronic derivation of the pressure signal.

Ad (5): Mean circumferential shortening velocity (MV_{CF}) can be calculated as follows

$$MV_{CF} = (LVEDD - LVESD) / (LVEDD \times LVET),$$

when LVEDD is the left ventricular end-diastolic diameter, LVESD is the left ventricular end-systolic diameter, and LVET is the left ventricular ejection time.

10.3. Results

Before the influence of either acute changes of myocardial energetics (positive inotropic compounds) or chronic changes of myocardial energetics (cardiac hypertrophy, ventricular dilatation, and heart failure) can be studied, the mechanical parameters, which determine myocardial oxygen consumption, must be defined.

10.3.1. Mechanical Parameters and Myocardial Oxygen Consumption

Heart rate is a very important and clear determinant of myocardial oxygen consumption. Therefore, in all our contributions regarding myocardial energetics, we analyzed the energy consumed by the myocardium for one heartbeat.

In a study investigating 19 subjects with normal left ventricular function and without any heart disease and 37 patients with dilated cardiomyopathy [15], we correlated measured myocardial oxygen consumption per beat to the respective mechanical parameters as there are:

(1) Systolic stress-time integral.
(2) Pressure-volume work.
(3) Peak systolic wall stress.
(4) dP/dt_{max}, i.e., maximum rate of pressure rise.
(5) MV_{CF}, i.e., mean velocity of circumferential shortening velocity.

The linear regression analysis of myocardial oxygen consumption per beat and the respective mechanical variables are shown in Table 1.

MVO_{2beat} as a function of STI					
N	0.90×STI	+	69.34	r=0.59	p<0.01
IDC	0.94×STI	+	37.25	r=0.65	p<0.001
MVO_{2beat} as a function of $\int P\cdot V$					
N	$2.64\times\int P\cdot V$	+	109.34	r=0.40	N.S.
IDC	$3.10\times\int P\cdot V$	+	109.13	r=0.33	p<0.05
MVO_{2beat} as a function of PSS					
N	0.22×PSS	+	87.75	r=0.39	N.S.
IDC	0.28×PSS	+	65.67	r=0.44	p<0.01
MVO_{2beat} as a function of dP/dt_{max}					
N	$-0.0003\times dP/dt_{max}$	+	138.92	r=0.01	N.S.
IDC	$0.014\times dP/dt_{max}$	+	125.97	r=0.11	N.S.
MVO_{2beat} as a function of MV_{CF}					
N	$-41.36\times MV_{CF}$	+	203.08	r=0.54	p<0.05
IDC	$8.70\times MV_{CF}$	+	135.22	r=0.06	N.S.

MVO_{2beat} myocardial oxygen consumption per beat; *STI* systolic stress-time integral; *$\int P\cdot V$* pressure-volume work; *PSS* peak systolic stress; *dP/dt_{max}* maximum rise of pressure development; *MV_{CF}* mean velocity of circumferential fiber shortening; *N* normal ventricles; *IDC* idiopathic dilated cardiomyopathy

Table 1: Linear regression analysis of myocardial oxygen consumption per beat and mechanical variables. According to [15].

From Table 1, it is quite clear that the only function, which holds true in both normal and dilated ventricles, is the MVO_2 vs. stress-time integral function. Although for other parameters a significant linear regression equation could be also found for either normal or dilated ventricles, the respective level of significance was always superior in case of the MVO_{2beat} vs. stress-time integral function. This finding is supported by the very early reports of Braunwald who established this index in the dog heart [16]. On the basis of these findings, we established the concept of myocardial energetics as analyzed in the human being in vivo by means of the relationship between oxygen consumption per beat and the systolic stress-time integral.

10.3.2. Alterations of Myocardial Energetics due to Acute Changes

In a number of studies, we investigated the following compounds with respect to changes in myocardial energetics in the human being in vivo:
(1) Sodium-nitroprusside, a strong vasodilator [17].
(2) Enoximone, a phosphodiesterase inhibitor [17].
(3) Xamoterol, a partial β_1-adrenoceptor agonist [18].
(4) Benazepril, an angiotensin-converting-enzyme inhibitor [19].
As a summary, the data are presented in Figure 5.

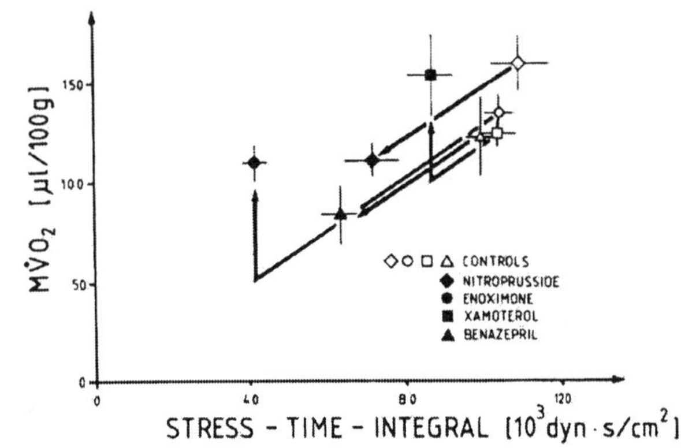

Figure 5: Myocardial oxygen consumption per beat (MVO_2) as a function of systolic stress-time-integral for 4 different pharmacological interventions: Pure vasodilators: Nitroprusside and ACE-inhibitor benazepril. Phosphodiesterase Inhibitor: Enoximone. Partial β_1-adrenoceptor agonist: Xamoterol.

From this diagram, it becomes clear that benazepril and nitroprusside, both venous and arteriolar vasodilators, reduce myocardial oxygen consumption due to a decrease in the systolic stress-time integral. Xamoterol having a positive inotropic effect via the b_1-adrenoceptor increases myocardial oxygen consumption when related to the respective stress-time integral. Enoximone has two effects: (1) It reduces the systolic stress-time integral by vasodilation of arteries and veins, but – due to myocardial stimulation via phosphodiesterase inhibition with subsequent increase in intracellular cyclic AMP – it increases MVO_{2beat} when related to the respective stress-time integral.

The "energy wasting effect" of enoximone via increase of cyclic AMP could also be demonstrated by correlation of MVO_2 to pressure-volume work or even better to pressure-volume-area as suggested by Suga and coworkers (see

Chapter IX). In Figure 6, the decrease in pressure-volume-area (PVA) is plotted as a function of the decrease in MVO_{2beat} due to application of sodium-nitroprusside and enoximone in two groups of patients suffering from dilated cardiomyopathy [17].

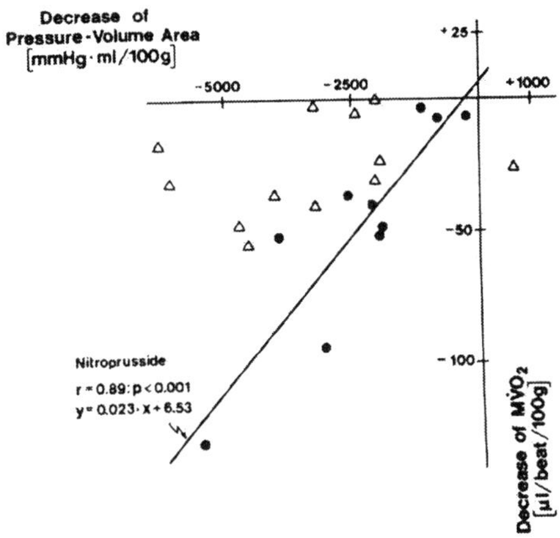

Figure 6: Decrease of PVA as a function of decrease in MVO_2: There is a clear correlation between these two parameters for conditions of nitroprusside [•] but not of emoximone [Δ].

A significant linear relationship could only be obtained for the intervention with sodium-nitroprusside. Under conditions of enoximone, however, the reduction of MVO_2 does not follow the reduction in PVA in 11 out of 12 treated patients indicating an "oxygen wasting effect" for this vasodilating and positive inotropic compound [17].

10.3.3. Alterations of Myocardial Energetics due to Chronic Changes

On the basis of a large number of patients with normal ventricles, hypertrophied ventricles due to aortic stenosis, and dilated ventricles due to idiopathic dilated cardiomyopathy, in which we have measured MVO_{2beat} as well as mechanical parameters, we are in a position to analyze myocardial energetics of hypertrophied and failing myocardium in comparison to normal myocardium.

10.3.3.1. The Failing vs. the Normal Heart

The failing heart is best described by the dilatation of the left chamber as demonstrated representatively in Figure 7: The left ventricular dimensions have greatly increased and, thereby, the ejection fraction is low despite a well maintained stroke volume at rest.

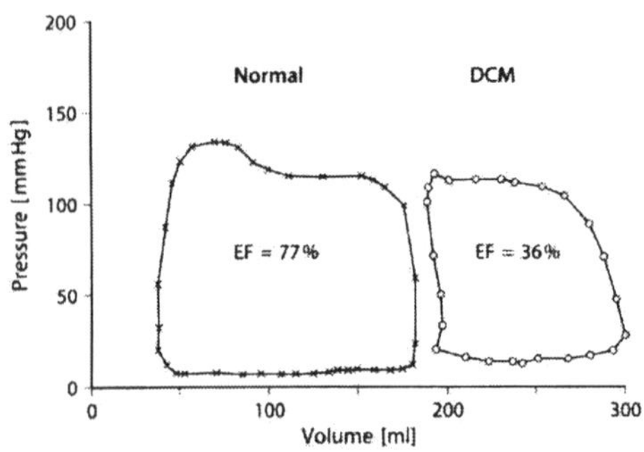

Figure 7: Pressure-volume relations for a normal and a dilated ventricle. Ejection fraction is given. DCM, dilated cardiomyopathy.

To compensate increased systolic wall stress, left ventricular hypertrophy develops: An increase of left ventricular wall mass from about 180 g to about 320 g (dilated) in our study population. It is important to note, however, that this kind of hypertrophy can almost normalize peak systolic wall stress but not at all the systolic stress-time integral. As shown in Figure 8 for two representative left ventricles (normal and dilated) and in Figure 9 for the whole study population, peak systolic stress is only 11 % higher in the dilated ventricles, whereas systolic stress-time integral is 44 % and thus significantly higher in dilated ventricles [15].

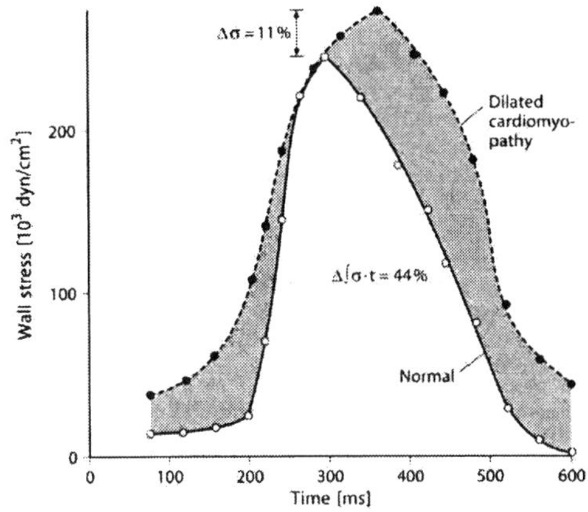

Figure 8: Systolic stress-time integrals for a normal and dilated ventricle. Whereas peak stress is greater in dilated ventricles by only 11%, systolic stress-time integral is increased by 42%. According to [15].

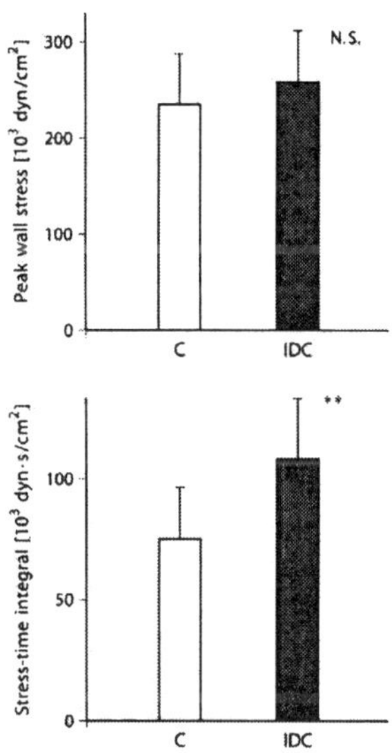

Figure 9: Peak systolic wall stress ***(upper columns)*** *and systolic stress-time integral* ***(lower columns)*** *in healthy individuals (C) and patients with dilated cardiomyopathy (IDC). ** $p < 0.001$. According to [15].*

Because MVO_{2beat} was virtually the same in normal and dilated ventricles, the quotient of the stress-time integral divided by MVO_{2beat}, which is an index of myocardial economy of contraction, is about 40 % higher in the failing myocardium.

In contrast, when we calculated myocardial efficiency, i.e., pressure-volume work divided by MVO_{2beat}, this index was greatly dependent on the enlargement of the ventricle, i.e., the larger the left ventricular end-diastolic volume, the lower the myocardial efficiency (Figure 10) [15].

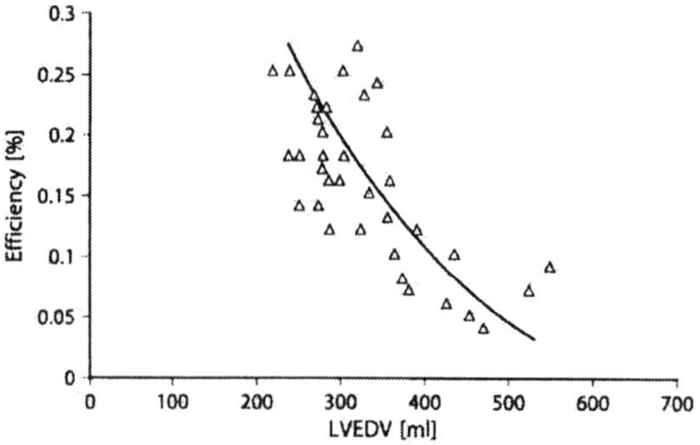

Figure 10: External efficiency as a function of left ventricular enddiastolic volume. A significant and inverse correlation was found. According to [15].

10.3.3.2. Hypertrophied vs. Normal Ventricles

We have also investigated myocardial energetics in patients suffering from severe aortic stenosis before they underwent aortic valve replacement surgery. In these hypertrophied ventricles, the relationship between MVO_{2beat} and systolic stress-time between MVO_{2beat} and systolic stress-time integral was significantly different from that obtained in normal ventricles indicating increased myocardial economy of hypertrophied myocardium (Figure 11).

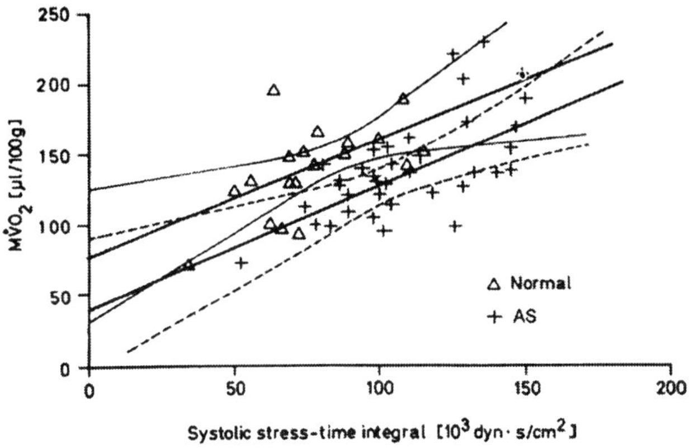

Figure 11: MVO_2 plotted versus stress-time integral in healthy individuals and patients with aortic stenosis (AS). Related to a unit of stress-time integral, MVO_2 is lower in cardiac hypertrophy due to aortic stenosis. Unpublished data.

Interestingly, in these hypertrophied but not dilated left ventricles, myocardial efficiency was not significantly different from that of normal left ventricles (no Figure).

10.4. Discussion

When an analysis of myocardial energetics is performed in the human being in vivo, it is necessary to measure myocardial oxygen consumption as well as mechanical parameters. The key for a proper description of myocardial energetics in vivo is (1) the calculation of myocardial oxygen consumption per beat (MVO_{2beat}) and (2) the correlation of MVO_{2beat} to the most important mechanical determinants of MVO_{2beat}. The calculation of MVO_2 for one cardiac cycle implies that the ration between MVO_{2beat} and mechanical variables is not substantially influenced by heart rate per se. Accordingly, Rooke and Feigl [20] demonstrated that myocardial oxygen consumption per beat is not influenced by heart rate when hemodynamic variables were kept constant.

In normal and in dilated ventricles, the best correlation was found for the function between MVO_{2beat} and systolic stress-time integral. Nevertheless, we also analyzed myocardial efficiency by taking pressure-volume work (area) into account (see also Chapter IX).

The data presented in this way clearly indicate that myocardial energetics are changed due to acute interventions and chronic mechanisms associated with cardiac hypertrophy and failure.

10.4.1. Acute Changes of Myocardial Energetics

Reduction of afterload alone by sodium-nitroprusside or reduction of both afterload and preload by benazepril, an angiotensin-converting-enzyme inhibitor, acutely lowers the systolic stress-time integral and thereby myocardial oxygen consumption as demonstrated in Figure 5. This reduction of MVO_{2beat} can only take place, because neither sodium-nitroprusside nor benzapril have acute stimulatory effects on left ventricular myocardium in the sense of an inotropic effect.

In contrast, substances that increase intracellular myocardial cyclic AMP levels either by stimulation of β_1-adrenoceptors (xamoterol) or by inhibition of phosphodiesterases (enoximone) clearly increase MVO_{2beat} when related to the respective stress-time integral. The "energy wasting effect" of enoximone can also be demonstrated when the pressure-volume area is used as mechanical determinant of myocardial oxygen consumption [17]. These data are in good agreement with experimental data discussed in chapter IV, V, and VI, although, from in vivo data, we cannot speculate on molecular mechanisms, i.e., calcium handling and cross-bridge kinetics.

10.4.2. Chronic Changes of Myocardial Energetics

There are at least three important observations in our investigations of myocardial energetics in hypertrophied and failing ventricles: (1) Geometrical factors, i.e., left ventricular dilation or remodeling, go hand in hand with a decrease of myocardial efficiency. Therefore, by therapeutic reduction of left ventricular size using either pharmacological or surgical tools myocardial efficiency may be improved. (2) In hypertrophied as well as failing human left ventricles MVO_{2beat} as related to systolic stress-time integral is reduced when compared to normal ventricles. These data are consistent with experimental animal data (see Chapter IV, V, and VI) and imply subtle molecular alterations of the human myocardium during hypertrophy and failure. These molecular changes may involve calcium handling proteins as well as contractile proteins. (3) In the compensated but failing human heart, cardiac hypertrophy, i.e., increase in left ventricular muscle mass and wall thickness, adjusts for normalization of peak systolic wall stress (Figure 8). Despite this compensatory mechanism, in the failing heart the stress-time integral was found to be increased compared to normal ventricles. There are two explanations for this increase in stress-time integral: (1) There are geometrical factors that may explain insufficient decrease of mechanical afterload of left ventricular myocardium at the end of systolic ejection period. (2) Altered molecular mechanisms involving reduced calcium handling and/or contractile protein interactions may be responsible. It is very likely that both mechanisms contribute to the observed biological phenomena.

REFERENCES

1) Bing RJ, Hammond MM, Handelman JC, Powers SR, Spencer FC, Eckenhoff JE, Goodale WT, Haffens HJ, Kety SS:The measurement of coronary blood flow, oxygen consumption and efficiency of the left ventricle in man. Am Heart J 1949;38:1-24

2) Kern MJ, Donohue ThJ: Evaluation of myocardial blood flow and metabolism. In: Cardiac Catheterization, Angiography, and Intervention. Eds: Baim DS, Grossmann W. Williams and Williams 1996;pp 359-389

3) Zeiher AM, Drexler H, Wollschläger H, Just H: Endothelial dysfunction of the coronary microvasculature is associated with impaired coronary flow regulation in patients with early atherosclerosis. Circulation 1991;84:1984-1992

4) Ganz W, et al.: Measurements of coronary sinus blood flow by continuous thermodilution in man. Circulation 1971;44:181-191

5) Baim DS, Rothman MT, Harrison DC: Improved catheter for regional coronary sinus flow and metabolic studies. Am J Cardiol 1980;46:997-1009

6) Kety SS, Schmidt CF: The nitrous oxide method for the quantitative determination of cerebral blood flow in man: Theory, procedure and normal values. J Clin Invest 1948;27:476-483

7) Bretschneider HJ, Gott L, Hilgert G, Probst R, Rau G: Gaschromatographische Trennung und Analyse von Argon als Basis einer neuen Fremdgasmethode zur Durchblutungsmessung von Organen. Verh Dtsch Ges Kreisl-Forsch 1966;32:267-273

8) Rau G: Messung der Koronardurchblutung mit der Argon-Fremdgas-methode. Arch Kreisl-Forschung 1969;58:322-398

9) Heiss HW, Blümchen G: Durchblutungsmessungen am Koronargefäßsystem. In: Reindell H, Roskamm H (eds): Herzkrankheiten. Springer Verlag Heidelberg New York 1982:pp 413-422

10) Sandler H, Dodge HT, Coble YD, Hay RE: The use of single plane angiocardiograms for the calculation of the left ventricular volume in man. Am Heart J 1968;75:

11) Rackley CE, Dodge HT, Coble YD, Hay RE: A method for determining left ventricular mass in man. Circulation 1964;29:666-671

12) v. Herrath M, Holubarsch Ch, Hasenfuss G, Heiss HW, Just H: Repeat determination of left ventricular wall thickness from mass and volume during one cardiac cycle. Clinical Cardiology 1990;13:218-220

13) Fifer MA, Grossmann W: Measurements of ventricular volumes, ejection fraction, mass, wall stress, and regional wall motion. In: Baim DS, Grossmann W (eds): Cardiac catheterization, angiography, and intervention. Williams and Williams 1996, Baltimore: pp 315-331

14) Mirsky I: Elastic properties of myocardium. A quantitative approach with physiological and clinical application. In: Berne RM (ed), Handbook of Physiology. The Cardiovascular System. Washington, DC, American Physiological Society 1979:497-531

15) Holubarsch ChJF: Geometrical considerations in (reverse) remodeling. In: Surgical Remodeling in Heart Failure. Brett W, Todoro A, Pfisterer M, Zerkowski HR (eds). Steinkopff-Verlag Darmstadt 2000:67-82

16) Sarnoff SJ, Braunwald E, Welch GH, Case RB, Stainsby WN, Macruz R: Hemodynamic determinants of oxygen consumption of the heart with special reference to the tension-time index. Am J Physiol 1958;192:148-162

17) Hasenfuss G, Holubarsch Ch, Heiss W, Meinertz Th, Bonzel T, Wais U, Lehmann M, Just H: Myocardial energetics in patients with dilated cardiomyopathy. Influence of nitroprusside and enoximone. Circulation 1989;80:51-64

18) Thierfelder L, Holubarsch Ch, Hasenfuss G, Heiss WH, Just H: The effect of the partial beta-1-adrenoceptor agonist xamoterol on hemodynamics and myocardial energetics in patients with dilated cardiomyopathy. J Cardiac Pharmacol 1991;17:593-599

19) Holubarsch Ch, Hasenfuss G, Thierfelder L, Just H: Energetic consequences of substances currently used or recommended for long-term treatment of chronic heart failure. In: Smith JFM (ed): Pharmacology of cardiac and vascular remodeling. Steinkopff Verlag Darmstadt 1991:107-112

20) Rooke CA, Feigl EO: Work as correlate of canine left ventricular oxygen consumption, and the problem of catecholamine oxygen wasting. Circ Res 1982;50:273-286

INDEX